THE YOGA OF SOUND

THE YOGA OF SOUND

Tapping the Hidden Power of Music and Chant

RUSSILL PAUL

FOREWORD BY WAYNE TEASDALE

NEW WORLD LIBRARY
NOVATO, CALIFORNIA

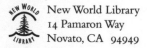

New World Library
14 Pamaron Way
Novato, CA 94949

The material in this book and the accompanying audio tracks is intended for education. It is not meant to take the place of diagnosis and treatment by a qualified medical practitioner or therapist. No expressed or implied guarantee as to the effects of the use of the recommendations can be given nor liability taken.

Text design: Cathey Flickinger

Kundalini illustration on page 86 used with permission of the Joseph Campbell Foundation (www.jcf.org).

Cover photo of Insight Yoga Studio, Pasadena, California

Library of Congress Cataloging-in-Publication Data
Paul, Russill.
The yoga of sound : tapping the hidden power of music and chant / Russill Paul.
p. cm.
Includes bibliographical references and index.
ISBN: 978-1-57731-536-0 (alk. paper)
1. Sound—Religious aspects—Hinduism. 2. Yoga. 3. Mantras. I. Title.
BL1215.S67P38 2004
294.5'37—dc22 2004004065

First paperback edition, April 2006
Originally published in hardcover in June 2004
ISBN: 978-1-57731-536-0
Printed in Canada on acid-free, partially recycled paper
Distributed to the trade by Publishers Group West

10 9 8 7 6 5

CONTENTS

PART 4: PRACTICE

The elements of Sound Yoga

PART 5: INTEGRATION

Living the life of a sound yogi

To Bede Griffiths, 1906–1993,
my spiritual father, mentor, and dear friend.
Your love and light shine through this work.

FOREWORD

Certain forms of music, like beautiful fragrances, awaken associations in us that are primordial, eternal, and ultimate. These timeless associations call us to the core of our spiritual being. They address something in us that cannot die or be corrupted, a yearning that reaches out to the infinite. This is sonic mysticism, a reality we can all encounter in our lives if we open ourselves to the experience. Sonic mysticism is the spirituality of sound expressing the Divine Reality. The Sufis say that some music grants us a faint experience of God, an echo of divine reality and presence. The Hindu tradition, in its practical understanding of sound in the mystical life, tells us that music *is* God when it reaches its ultimate purity, focus, and effectiveness in opening the heart, mind, and spirit.

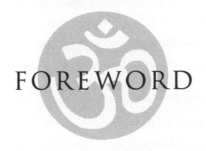

Music and sound permeate the cosmos — perhaps all universes and realms, including Heaven itself. Experiments in the physics of acoustics have demonstrated that sound affects reality by actually creating structure. Using radio telescopes, astronomers have found sound throughout every corner of the universe. They have also discovered that some of the haunting sounds that inspire our most sacred music in many traditions are actually cosmic sonic elements, the sounds of the universe itself. This astounding discovery suggests how intimately we are connected with the cosmic matrix, and how deeply it affects us all.

It is also clear from consciousness studies that music, chant, and sound have direct and dramatic effects on consciousness. It doesn't take much to realize how profound a role music often plays in our lives. The sonic principle is indispensable to the full development of the human, particularly in relation to the mystical journey — the moral, intellectual, psychological, and spiritual evolution of individuals, communities, nations, and the entire human family.

An angel holding a violin once appeared to St. Francis of Assisi. As the angel ran the bow very slowly over the strings, the heavenly music emanating from the instrument sent the saint into an intense ecstasy. Many of us have had similar mystical experiences. I remember listening to an angelic piece of music by David Hykes's Harmonic Choir. Having received the CD as a Christmas gift, I opened it just before retiring one evening and reclined in my favorite chair. I cannot say what happened, except that it propelled me to a mystical state that is impossible to describe. It literally took me beyond this world! Such is the spiritual power of music.

Russill Paul's *The Yoga of Sound* relates to these experiences, but really it is an entirely unique work in a class all its own. There are hundreds of books on yoga, and some of them are outstanding, but this book is a pioneering achievement in sonic mysticism. Russill has been my dear friend for many years. We shared a common spiritual guide in Bede Griffiths, and we first developed our friendship in the monsastic community of Shantivanam ashram in south India eighteen years ago. We continue to enjoy a spiritual brotherhood through collaborative practice and teaching into the present day.

Knowing him as I do, I will not hesitate to identify Russill as a musical and spiritual genius, and this book is evidence of his gifts. Coming from the Indian tradition of Sound Yoga, a decisively contemplative means of achieving integration with the Divine, Russill's writing and work stand on the shoulders of giants going back thousands of years. No other tradition has gone further, deeper, and higher than the Indian in exploring sound as a mystical method of union with the Absolute. This entire Indian body of spiritual wisdom has many strands. The West has embraced the physical strand of Hatha Yoga, but most of the other strands remain unknown in the West. This brilliant but very accessible and practical book illuminates not only the sonic element but how the many strands of yoga tradition fit together.

As a master of sonic mysticism, Russill has developed his own synthesis of this profoundly rich and effective tradition. He has assimilated this tradition through his intense study and contemplative life, and he has discovered a way to articulate it in terms intelligible to Western culture. Russill makes a very persuasive case for incorporating this sonic science into the Western practice of yoga. This is a remarkable achievement, and one that didn't come easy. Russill's understanding of the needs of the American culture and its great diversity, along with his knowledge of how much this sonic dimension can enrich our culture, have been his constant motivations. He has given us the gift of Sound Yoga as a spiritual practice, until now a barely discovered means to enlightenment.

Samadhi, one of the goals of the Yoga of Sound, is an infinite, pure consciousness that transcends the vagaries of time. This pure consciousness, the nondual reality we all share as our deeper nature, is the destiny of sonic mysticism. In bringing about this emergence into pure consciousness, the Yoga of Sound, as Russill points out, is "an alchemy of the soul." Although this practice will facilitate healing and relaxation, Russill shows us that arriving at, and dwelling in, pure consciousness is its final purpose. This purpose requires us to know the fullness of immortal, pure, and immutable consciousness — our common ground and the basis of our reality.

Russill's book fills an important need in third millennial spirituality. Until now, there has been very little to represent this dimension of spiritual life in Western mystical studies and practical discipline. Doubtless the publication of this volume will inspire others of its type, but it would be very hard to equal what has been accomplished in these pages. This book is a new classic in both yoga and spirituality. Its impact will be felt around the world for ages to come.

Wayne Teasdale
Chicago, Illinois
March 2004

PREFACE TO THE PAPERBACK EDITION

Every culture has its own form of sonic mysticism. Gospel music manifests the spiritual power of sound, as do symphony orchestras, Hebrew cantors, Sufi Qawwali singers, Siberian shamans, Benedictine monks, and the Tibetan Gyuto choir. But yoga comes from India, and since sound, in the form of mantra, has shared a close partnership with the postures and gestures of yoga over many millennia of evolution, the Yoga of Sound draws its insights and practices essentially from the Hindu tradition of yoga and meditation. Readers steeped in the practice of mantra or knowledgeable about Hindu spirituality may consider the term *the Yoga of Sound* nontraditional. Well, it is and it isn't. I use *the Yoga of Sound* to denote the entire scope of sacred sound that developed within traditional Hinduism and the broad context of yoga. It offers anyone on the path of yoga, or for that matter anyone interested in the spiritual power of sound, insights into the yogic possibilities of vocalization in the service of higher consciousness.

Yoga is essentially the refining of consciousness. This book is an effort to create a holistic and evolutionary approach to a rapidly growing interest in Sanskrit mantra and the widespread use of chanting as a spiritual practice in the Western world. Chanting is not a New Age fad; the use of sound as a means of yoga is grounded in traditions thousands of years old. While Mantra Yoga, Japa Yoga, and kirtan denote parts or aspects of the process, the term *the Yoga of Sound* seeks to embrace all of these possibilities and more.

The official term for the use of sound and music as a spiritual path is *Nada Yoga*, which literally translates as "Sound Yoga." In this sense, Nada Yoga, or Sound Yoga, with its impressive two-thousand-year documented history, is as formidable as Hatha Yoga, the popular yoga of postures, stretches, and breathing techniques practiced widely today. One might easily assume that all forms of mantra are included in Nada Yoga. Interestingly, however, the practice of Nada Yoga, as described in numerous texts, focuses mostly on the syllable Om, along with various listening practices. Later, with the development of Indian music, particularly in the Middle Ages, Nada Yoga began to involve the use of language in musical form but still did not truly position the sophisticated technology of mantra as integral to the refining of consciousness. Etymologically, *Nada* is sound in the form of pitch, tone, and drone, while *Shabda* is sound in the form of word, meaning, and language.

Therefore, rather than title this book *Nada Yoga*, or *Sound Yoga*, I use *the Yoga of Sound* to present all the major streams of sacred sound prevalent in Hinduism: through the Vedic tradition's knowledge-based Gnostic schools, the Tantric tradition's body-based yogic schools, and the Bhakti tradition's ecstatic cults of devotion. All these traditions go back thousands of years, and the role of sound is well documented within each of them. But because sound, in and of itself, is capable of awakening deep states of mystical consciousness that lead to healing and spiritual transformation, sound itself is a legitimate "yoga," or path, with its own unique capabilities for mystical union and self-realization. This is a condition described in numerous sacred sound texts and something you can easily discover for yourself through practicing the downloadable audio exercises.

Nada Yoga, in the way I have presented it in this work, is treated as a unique stream of sacred sound, with its own specific qualities. Following suit, I have chosen to present mantra from the Vedic tradition under the term *Shabda Yoga*, because the Vedas are essentially based on the spiritual power of the word (shabda). Similarly, I have used the term *Shakti Yoga* to describe the application of sound and mantra drawn from the Tantric tradition, since the goal of Tantra is to transform energy (shakti) from gross to subtle through the spiritual alchemy of Tantric yoga. Likewise, I have used the term *Bhava Yoga* to present the use of mantra and other sacred sound practices, including kirtan and japa, from the Bhakti tradition. (*Bhava* is spiritual feeling, the predisposition toward devotional yoga.) Each of these streams has been isolated in the past, at least in the sense that one could not actually study them all in one place. Here, we have a more accessible, meaningful, and personalized expression of sacred sound from the classic Vedic, Tantric, and Bhakti traditions.

Under the auspices of these four streams of sacred sound — Shabda Yoga, Shakti Yoga, Bhava Yoga, and Nada Yoga — I have tried to present the Yoga of Sound as an integrated system through which specific mantras can be studied within the context of each stream's particular styles, applications, functions, and vocal methods. The Yoga of Sound also serves to encourage the application of mantras in relationship to other components of yoga, rather than as a stand-alone practice. Thus, the Yoga of Sound requires bringing five different components together: sound, posture, breath, movement, and consciousness. When we effectively combine all these components, yoga happens!

This book will give you a good sense of what is possible and how you can apply the vast traditions of mantra to your life today. The Yoga of Sound, as a system, provides an extensive vocabulary of spiritual practices and sounds that, when properly learned, enables the practitioner to work with the rapidly changing dynamics of modern life, helping us realize that we are not alone and that we are not without power. I will show how mantras can be used to access the energy, power, and intelligence we need at any moment or in any circumstance, not through some cookie-cutter approach, but through an open system that can be tailor-made to each of our needs, allowing us to take control of our energy and then channel it effectively into our professions, our relationships, and most of all, into our spiritual progress. Mantra is, after all, a means to an end, and that end is wholeness.

Obviously, the Yoga of Sound intersects with many traditional forms of yoga: Hatha Yoga, Kundalini Yoga, Bhakti Yoga, and so on. (In fact, most of Hinduism's traditional schools draw from a variety of sources; they are not as mutually exclusive as we are often led to believe. Even the distinct Vedic, Tantric, and Bhakti traditions cross over into one another.) The Yoga of Sound should therefore be viewed as an evolving paradigm that combines mantra with other forms of yogic practice, particularly with ritual, an aspect of healing with which we are fast losing touch. Mantra originally developed within the context of ritual, which is something we may have to reinvent for ourselves today.

Ultimately, the Yoga of Sound should reach beyond the confines of traditional Hinduism to embrace all the spiritual traditions of the world, advancing knowledge in science, medicine, and all viable means of healing and enlightenment. I offer the Yoga of Sound therefore as a postmodern term, as a means of bringing together the ancient wisdom of our yogic ancestors with modern technology and then innovatively applying it to modern lifestyles. The extraordinary advances of our recording and audio technologies can and should be used for higher spiritual purposes, assisting us in opening the doors of our mystical perception and awakening powerful energies of transformation for our species. This is the future of spiritual practice. Welcome to the world of sacred sound.

ACKNOWLEDGMENTS

I thank my editor, Jason Gardner, who has lovingly helped shape the content of this book into its present form; kudos also to Carol Venolia for her razor-sharp copyediting and many helpful suggestions. Much gratitude is due to my wife Asha, who is also my best friend and beloved playmate. What a gift! I thank my parents Anthony and Josephine for the immense freedom and love they gave me, and my sister Marlene for her many literary influences. Special thanks go to my in-laws, the Muthayah family, for their unconditional love and faith in me.

I thank Paul Winter, Carlos Santana, Mozart, and all the other musical icons who have influenced my world of sound through their genius. Special thanks go to Arlo Guthrie for his spiritual presence and loving support. I offer my deepest respect to all my teachers of yoga, music, and Sanskrit.

I extend my heartfelt thanks to my dear friend Diane Kelliger, who was also my business advisor and moral support for many years; her dedication to spiritual practice and a healthy lifestyle never ceases to amaze and inspire me. Much gratitude is due to Andre Poirier, who has been a loving godfather and a great source of comfort throughout my life in the West. I also thank my friends Margy and Jim Gresham for investing unconditionally in my art. I thank Wayne Teasdale for his tremendous faith in me as a writer and for all his assistance to me over the years as friend, mentor, spiritual brother, and literary inspiration; we go back a long way.

I thank Matthew Fox for his love of my artistry, his friendship, and his devotion to recovering the sacred in art. I thank my students of the past twenty years. Without them, this work could not have developed as it has. I thank the institutions that have allowed me to teach this work, particularly the graduate department of Naropa University in Oakland, California, and the Doctor in Ministry program of the University of Creation Spirituality, also in Oakland. Last but not least, I thank my devoted fans and well-wishers.

INTRODUCTION

Life has a vital sonic dimension that colors our moods and sentiments, our joys and fears, our love and pain. Without the energy and emotion that sound and music provide, our lives would feel disembodied — even dead. As you reflect on your life, you will realize that significant events have often been preceded by a sense of music in the air, informing you that something wonderful was about to unfold. The opposite is equally true: An ominous silence or an atmosphere darkened by dissonant sound often foretells a coming disaster. For those who have developed their ears to hear more intently, a wealth of information is available to guide them through the diversity of life's experiences. It is the power of this subtle sonic dimension that we seek to master through the Yoga of Sound.

I wrote this book to introduce an ancient yet almost unknown practice to those who want to broaden and deepen the spiritual dimension of their lives. The personal benefits I have enjoyed via the Yoga of Sound have been immense. It works. Over the past twenty years, the students with whom I've shared this tradition have also experienced its benefits. Yet a comprehensive, reader-friendly understanding of the role of sound in yoga practice is not presently available in the West. In this book, I want to make the depth and scope of Sound Yoga accessible to anyone who is interested in using sound and music as a spiritual practice.

You might wonder if you need to be musical to embark on this journey. You don't need to be musical, but you will find yourself becoming more musical as your practice develops. How is sound different from music? Sound is the emanation of any tone, frequency, or vibration. Quantum physicists tell us that in order for anything to exist it has to be in motion, vibrating. Conversely, if any object is in motion, it is producing a frequency — a specific tone. Refrigerators, airplanes, automobiles, and hair dryers all produce tones. Your body, too, exists because every atom and cell in your organism is vibrating. Life is vibration, tone, and rhythm. In this sense, everything is alive. Music, on the other hand, is the organization of specific tones or frequencies, located at specific distances — or musical intervals — from each other. Sound is always implicit in music. But when we think of sound as vibration, we can understand that the scope of all the vibrating frequencies in the universe goes far beyond the range of what our human ears can hear. Music is the perception and understanding of the underlying order and relationships among all these vibrations, expressed in melody, rhythm, and harmony. Even our sense of music may be rather limited in relation to its possibilities in our mysterious universe.

In today's world, sounds of varying quality often overwhelm us. We have become accustomed to the barrage of sound in our cars, homes, elevators, stores, and public spaces. This onslaught is corroding our emotional taste buds and destroying our capacity to sense the finer shades of existence. A CompuServe news survey in December 2002 found that roughly one-fifth of Americans felt that loud noise made their lives stressful. And unhealthy stress, we now know, is a key precipitator of disease. "So sensitive are we to sound that noise pollution has been called the most common modern health hazard," writes alternative physician Dr. Larry Dossey. "High levels of unpleasant sounds cause blood vessels to constrict; increase the blood pressure, pulse, and respiratory rates; release extra fats into the bloodstream; and cause the blood's magnesium level to fall."[1]

These effects don't come as a surprise to most of us; we all tolerate a lot of noise. But how effectively are we compensating for this intrusion? The answer lies in the highs and lows of our emotions and spirit. If we are swinging toward the extremes, then we are probably not coping well with the effects of this invasion of unhealthy sound.

When we look within our bodies, we discover another world of sound — one that feels the influence of our increasingly noisy exterior world. Heartbeats, nerve twitches, and the blinking of our eyes all emit vibrations, and these inner vibrations are being entrained to those generated by the outer world. Entrainment is the process by which natural motions become synchronized, such as the pendulums of clocks or the menstrual cycles of women who live in community. Even two heart-muscle cells pulsing at different rates will start to pulse together if brought into proximity of each other. In the same way, when our outer world is cacophonic, that discordant vibration will configure our inner world. Conversely, inner turmoil manifests as a manic outer world. How can we learn to shift this process? How do we create a more harmonious inner world, which then improves our outer world? This is exactly what we will explore through the Yoga of Sound.

When we fall out of harmony with ourselves or our world — when we are nervous, afraid, or unhappy — our inner sounds become discordant and we don't feel well. In ancient Greece, medicine was used to keep the body in tune — in harmonic alignment with nature and the universe. All forms of sickness, both physical and mental, were considered musical inconsistencies. Hippocrates, the father of Western medicine, often took his patients to the healing temple of Asclepius. There, music was used to reestablish the natural harmony of the body. Compare this to our modern hospitals, where noxious, hazardous sounds are ubiquitous. Patients recovering from heart attacks in coronary care units, for instance, are particularly susceptible to unpleasant sounds, and noise pollution in these settings can affect survival and recovery. [2]

The Yoga of Sound counteracts noise pollution; it helps us establish and maintain the natural harmony of our bodies. It is a spiritual practice that shows us how to work with all the sound in our lives, giving us the discernment to separate the good from the bad and empowering us to weave it all into one harmonious fabric.

In today's environments, managing stress has become the primary factor in maintaining our health and well-being. Yet stress is a necessary component of our productive lives; few of us want to return to living in the woods or sitting in a cave just to escape stress. We want to fully engage with the world, and at the same time we want a spiritual life that will help us cope with stress.

No matter how exciting our lives may be, we feel that something is missing if we don't touch the deeper parts of ourselves. We thus feel compelled to move inward, into the core of our being, to discover the true nature of our soul in the rapidly changing landscape of our thoughts and emotions. Balancing these inward and outward impulses seems to call for a sort of guerrilla spirituality — something we can practice without giving up the world. The Yoga of Sound, an ancient and well-tested discipline, can be that practice.

MY JOURNEY

I FIRST DISCOVERED the Yoga of Sound when I officially renounced the world at the age of nineteen. The process of renunciation took about a year to unfold; when I was sure, I called my family together in our home in South India and declared that I was going to join an ashram. I had grown up in a Christian family, and my mother was appalled; she imagined that I was going to team up for group sex at the local Rajneesh center, the only kind of "ashram" she knew about. But I had my heart set on Shantivanam, a peaceful oasis on the banks of the holy river Cauvery. There, in the shade of the eucalyptus and mango trees, I discovered an amazing way of life based on chanting, meditation, and yoga.

The monastery I joined was a Benedictine ashram, a Hindu-Christian hybrid directed by Bede Griffiths, an English Benedictine monk who had moved to India to explore Eastern spirituality. Under his direction, a whole world of interior sound opened for me. Ever since I'd been a young boy, I had aspired to be a professional musician. I had trained myself in rock, jazz, and pop, hoping to perform with the world's great artists (Carlos Santana was one of my favorites). But in the ashram, my awareness of sound was expanded. Through many wonderful teachers around the great temples of South India, I learned about the sacredness of music in the Indian *Carnatic* tradition. I also studied ancient Sanskrit chanting and began to read sacred Hindu texts about exploring consciousness through sound and music. I was thrilled to discover a practice that combined my love of music with my spiritual search.

Five years after joining the ashram, I married Asha, who had also lived at Shantivanam. Together we came to the West, intending to explore sound and music within the context of healing and spirituality. We chose North America because of the rapidly growing interest in yoga here, as well as the developing acceptance of therapeutic music.

Life in the West taught me about the true value of the Yoga of Sound, which can effectively bring much-needed balance to the lifestyle here. I found myself rediscovering the sacred in a culture that was the exact opposite of what I'd experienced in India. Modern America is radically different from modern India, which retains a strong sense of the sacred in public places and professional environments. Waving incense in front of a sacred image before a studio recording, or breaking coconuts ceremoniously at the start of a movie, are just two of countless reminders of the sacred in the daily life of present-day Indians.

Yet America is not without its own spiritual power, so I want to be respectful of this culture as I introduce my knowledge of Eastern spirituality here. The first wave of Indian teachers sought to transplant Hindu spirituality, unchanged, into Western soil. I believe that a new attitude is necessary today. The insights I will share with you through the Yoga of Sound are offered in a spirit of dialogue and sensitive cross-cultural fertilization. I hope that this effort will, in some fashion, enrich the global spiritual renaissance that is taking root here in the West.

The practice of Hatha Yoga has recently exploded in the West, as people enjoy the flexibility, health, and stress reduction it offers the body. With this book, I hope to educate and motivate Western yoga practitioners (yogis) to also incorporate sacred sound into their practice. A better education about this sonic science will allow American yogis to expand the scope of yogic states available to them.

At present, the practice of Sound Yoga in America is almost entirely limited to devotional chanting, or *kirtan* — a call-and-response chant sung in praise of the Divine. Although devotional chanting is accessible and touches the heart quickly — two qualities that strongly attract the average practitioner — it is only one of four streams of sacred sound in yoga and Hinduism. If the world were all heart, devotional chanting would suffice for our sonic spirituality. But this is not the case, so limiting our sonic practice to kirtan leaves us poorly equipped to face our turbulent times. Through a varied, integrated sonic mysticism, we can discover strength, sensuality, and attunement, as well as devotion.

WHO BENEFITS?

After almost twenty years of teaching Westerners, I have found that an integrated practice that includes all four sonic streams appeals to many people. While the most obvious candidates for this path may appear to be yoga practitioners, the word "yogi" actually embraces any serious spiritual seeker who consciously and methodically aspires to achieve harmony, balance, and refined consciousness.

Mantras are the sounds that should accompany our yoga postures. Like strands of DNA, these sounds offer yoga practitioners a direct link to the source and substance of the yoga tradition. Just as you cannot truly grasp science without knowing its language — mathematics — it is impossible to touch upon the depth of yoga without a knowledge of mantras. Ranging from single, resonating syllables to long, recited sentences, mantras are the soul of the yoga tradition. Yoga practice fueled by an extensive vocabulary of mantras can effect profound spiritual awakenings. The time has arrived for yoga practitioners in the West to take this element seriously, and through it to discover their spiritual roots.

The Yoga of Sound has much to offer others as well. If you are not a yoga practitioner, but are inclined toward practices such as Tai Chi, Chi Gong, or forms of dance rather than yoga postures, you will find that the practice of mantra can increase your concentration, enhance your creativity, and enable you to maintain a healthy body and mind.

Health-care workers and people who seek healing for themselves will discover that the Yoga of Sound provides tools that connect them with the spiritual dimension of the healing process. Furthermore, research shows that chanting produces natural painkillers, lowers the heart rate, and reduces blood pressure — a few of many positive effects of sound on the body. The Yoga of Sound cannot replace medicine, but it certainly can augment it. Mantra has always been central to healing in India, where sonic formulas have been used to promote well-being for thousands of years. When used in combination with ritual, meditation, and Hatha Yoga practice, mantras become vessels of healing energy that we can direct within ourselves or into others.

For those interested in spiritual experience, the Yoga of Sound presents a tremendous range of practices that directly embody spiritual growth. You do not need to give up an existing practice or tradition to explore this path.

For artists, the Yoga of Sound offers a spiritual discipline that instills self-confidence, reconnects one with one's body, and helps clear creative blocks. Singers can add power to their art by widening the scope of their vocal and chanting abilities; through proper application of the Yoga of Sound, they can enjoy improved vocal texture, control, depth, and resonance. Indeed, any musician who discovers the language, cosmology, and spiritual technology behind the Yoga of Sound tradition will channel greater transformational energy into the world through their art and person.

And, of course, any busy person caught up in the frantic pace of the modern world can use the Yoga of Sound to relax, reduce stress, and awaken creative potential in new ways. Sound Yoga is an easy, effective way to still the chatter of the mind. The Yoga of Sound can also help people overcome addiction, a common result of excessive stress. Exploring the Yoga of Sound is about taking charge of our lives and our environments, and transforming them through spiritual practice.

Many of us are emotionally fragile and spiritually vulnerable. Energy constantly drains from numerous ruptures in our energy systems. As we develop our capabilities with the Yoga of Sound, we can gather both the pleasant and unpleasant energies we encounter and use them to our advantage, rather than being victimized by them. Imagine what a blessing it would be — and what a storehouse of power we would build — if we could convert the energy that flows through the many facets of our being into a positive force. The Yoga of Sound helps us harness the energy around and within us so that we can use it to transform our lives.

We have within us the power, the resources, and the skills to draw into our consciousness the experiences we value, moving us naturally toward a harmonious future. In this book, I will share with you the techniques I have used to make my own life increasingly harmonious. Grounded in traditions thousands of years old, the Yoga of Sound can be a powerful tool to transform your life and your world.

THE STRUCTURE OF THIS BOOK

Part one, "Yoga," deals with understanding both sound and yoga in a broad, deep sense. I will also discuss how the Yoga of Sound relates to, differs from, and complements Hatha Yoga. In part two, "Mantra," I will extensively address the subject of mantra, which is the language of yogic experience. In part three, "Tradition," I look at the four streams of sonic mysticism: *Shabda Yoga, Shakti Yoga, Bhava Yoga,* and *Nada Yoga.* I will further discuss the function and significance of various kinds of mantras within the context of these four streams and styles of Sound Yoga. The Yoga of Sound, as I am offering it you, is an integration of these four streams. In part four, I have broken down the practice of the Yoga of Sound into five elements: posture, the breath, sound, movement, and consciousness. Finally, in part five I will show you how to implement the knowledge you've gained through this work into a daily practice and continue your exploration of this amazing path.

Since the pronunciation of mantras is important, I have devised a simple method to train you in this aspect of chanting. Your experience of pronunciation will gradually unfold through the four appendixes included at the end of this book. These appendixes pertain to the four distinct streams of sonic mysticism mentioned earlier. However, I have not utilized this pronunciation system in regard to the Hindu terms I use throughout the book, choosing instead the common spellings that most readers are familiar with.

The accompanying audio tracks can help you experience and practice the four streams of Sound Yoga. To further expand your understanding, I have also included a section on programs and resources after the appendixes.

My vision of this work is to help you, first and foremost, grasp the depth and scope of this sonic mysticism. Next, I will reveal how useful this tradition is to our present-day lifestyles and challenges. Finally, I want to introduce you to the practical methods and techniques of this tradition. To that end, I provide you with exercises throughout the book, carefully described so that you can understand and practice them easily. You can also cross-reference specific practices by making use of the index; page numbers listed in boldface will help you locate where you can learn a given practice or mantra.

I hope you will enjoy the ride.

Namaste,
Russill Paul

PART 1

YOGA

A WAY OF HARMONY, BALANCE, AND ECSTASY

The Yogi, whose mind is in harmony, finds rest in the spirit within and deep communion with the whole universe. Free from restlessness her soul is like a lamp whose flame burns steady in a shelter where no winds blow.

Bhagavad Gita VI: 16–21

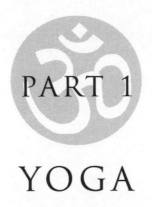

CHAPTER 1

BALANCING VISION AND SOUND

The human species suffers from a pervading imbalance because the eye dominates the ear, which corresponds to male forms dominating the female. Many of our problems, ranging from unrest in our relationships to international conflicts, can be minimized through reevaluating the way we view, utilize, and relate to sound — and, consequently, to the feminine in our lives. The Yoga of Sound can help us find balance for ourselves, our communities, and our world.

Much of the information we rely on comes to us through our eyes. This information can be measured, analyzed, and categorized — all processes of the linear left brain, also known as the masculine brain. To be successful in our society, we develop the left brain — often to the neglect of the right brain, which coordinates the artistic, intuitive, and feminine aspects of awareness. From the time when we wake up on a workday until we go to sleep at night, we must continually jerk ourselves into the analytical, organizing power of the left brain. Like the edge of a Neanderthal's spear, we must keep our left brain sharp throughout the day to provide for our families and defend ourselves from the predators of modern civilization. If we lapse into the artistic feminine brain, we might lose our ability to drive a car, cross a road, get money from an ATM, or communicate in a business meeting. Even our weekends and holidays, filled with the efficient execution of tasks and lists, are dominated by left-brain activities; we are constantly sifting through our options.

The left brain is about *doing;* the right brain is about *being.* One of our greatest difficulties these days is getting our linear, thinking mind to take a break. For instance, preoccupation with a problem, anxiety about an approaching outcome, or depression resulting from a difficult relationship can take over our mind and emotions. Harmonizing the flow of our thought patterns creates spaciousness in the mind and gives us perspective on our thought processes.

The main reason for taking vacations is that our feminine mind is starved most of the year. We only rest in the feminine mind when we eat, have sex, or sleep — and many of us have trouble sleeping because the left brain won't let go. The feminine mind relishes experience and takes in the whole rather than objectifying a part. All too often, we find that our thinking, describing mind invades and violates our moments of experiential absorption, diminishing even the short periods we set aside for ourselves.

"Yoga is *chitta vritti nirodha,*" begins Patanjali's famous set of aphorisms known as *The Yoga Sutras.*[1] In English, this means that yoga is the cessation of the movements and modifications of the mind. Present-day spiritual teacher Eckhart Tolle, author of *The Power of Now,*[2] has eloquently demonstrated this primary yogic principle by awakening people to the "off switch" that stops the thinking mind — or at least gives it a short rest. When we turn off that switch, the feminine mind is allowed to function and we find balance in our lives.

Here is another way of looking at these two forms of mind, which are represented by the two hemispheres of our brain. Typically, the left brain is governed by the ego, which is geared toward achievement, success, and doing. The right brain, on the other hand, is governed by the soul, which is engaged in processes for their own sake, without judgment of any kind. Since the right brain is free from the desire for specific outcomes, the soul can delight in the experience of *being.*

The Yoga of Sound is concerned primarily with the recovery and reconstitution of soul energy. And, as Western yogis seek to develop their own unique identity, the role of yogic music, sacred sound, and mantra is crucial to the soul of yoga as it develops in the West.

STRESS AND THE IMBALANCE OF THE VISUAL

Not only do external pressures cause us stress, but getting stuck in the left brain exacerbates that stress. Unfortunately, for most Americans television has become the standard way to relax and control stress. While television can help us relax and unwind after a long, hard day at work, it also bombards us with a tremendous amount of negative information that concentrates fear and anxiety in our bodies. Michael Moore's brilliant documentary *Bowling for Columbine* demonstrates how American television creates a culture of fear that is completely out of proportion with healthy caution.

Excessive television watching also reduces our attention span because we become conditioned to expect an unnatural level of stimulus and variety. This becomes a major barrier to spiritual development because the effects of healthy spiritual practice are often subtle and can go unnoticed by someone whose senses are overstimulated. Furthermore, the rapid segues from one scene to another in many television and movie productions, together with the onslaught of aggressive advertising, translate directly into our disembodied, disjointed lifestyles. This lack of continuity in our consciousness contributes to the ease with which we are drawn into the drama of the ego. Layers of stress build on each other, leading us to become quick in our judgments, which then contribute to a deepening skepticism, especially around spiritual practices. Such patterns have got to change if we are to find meaning, balance, and fulfillment in our lives.

Although we do our best to compensate for the imbalance between our left and right brains, we find that unresolved energy tends to accumulate. This accumulated energy can cause discomfort and blockage, or it can spill out in undesirable ways, often embarrassing us and harming our relationships. Many of these energy problems are subtle and unconscious, while others are more visible: sudden outbursts of anger, irrational fears, dejection, a sense of isolation and loneliness, and even deep depression that comes on without warning. When we fail to harmonize our emotions, and when we lack the means to properly release accumulated energy, these conditions eventually lead to discomfort, disease, and, in the worst cases, death.

Through the proper and systematic application of Sound Yoga, many of these conditions can be monitored and managed effectively, creating more desirable life situations and better health. Dr. Dharma Singh Khalsa, a medical expert and yogi, informs us that yogic mantras stimulate the secretions of the pituitary gland, which is located only millimeters from the palate. These secretions strengthen our immune and neurological systems, protecting us from disease and negative emotions. In various clinical and therapeutic applications, chanting has been found to control the production of stress hormones and increase the production of endorphins, the body's natural painkillers. Thus, there is also a physiological benefit from the use of sound as a yoga practice.

On a deeper level, the voice serves as a barometer of the soul's condition, reflecting our fears, anxieties, and negative emotions as well as our joys and strengths. Through conscious development of the voice, we can affect our body's chemical, psychological, and spiritual experiences. The Yoga of Sound generates a unifying power that allows us to experience life as a seamless piece of music with varying themes and textures. We learn to fulfill each of these themes as we move on to new ones, resulting in better resolution of our life experiences.

As we learn to combine authentic relaxation and balance with the right kind of energy stimulation, we will soon be on the road to true health and happiness. To get started on this journey, we must first understand how we treat and respect the power of the eye in relation to the power of the ear.

THE EYE AND EAR AS SYMBOLS OF POWER

IT DOESN'T TAKE MUCH to notice that art classes are the first to be cut in our education system, that intuitive responses often draw scorn in our professional environments, and that — despite our sophistication — insensitive and derogatory clichés about the female sex continue to plague our language. Art and intuition are both strongly generated by the right brain, which we consider feminine. To rectify this condition, we must recover our capacity to be a listening people. German musicologist

Joachim-Ernst Berendt argues that we, as a species, are suffering from "ocular hypertrophy" — an exaggerated and unnecessary growth and complexity of our visual function. Hypertrophy results from excessive nutrition. In this case, the "nutrition" is the rational, analytical knowledge received by the eyes.

In Berendt's inspirational work *The World Is Sound, Nada Brahma,* he explains that, in ancient indigenous cultures, the eye was symbolized by an arrow. The eye and the masculine brain are strongly connected; the eye sights its target and, like an arrow, speeds toward its object, violently penetrating it. The eagle's eye, which is seen as the ultimate development of this faculty, can observe from a distance, focus on a single part of its prey, capture the animal, then dissect and consume the part. This is exactly how the eye, as well as the egoic "I," approaches and absorbs knowledge: by tearing it apart and consuming it.

The ear, in ancient cultures, was associated with the conch shell, which also resembles the gateway to the female reproductive organs. The ear is feminine and soul-like because of its receptive, deep, interior, mysterious qualities. This is why the quality of our hearing and the kinds of sounds we hear are important; we derive healing and nourishment for our soul from the process. In other words, to neglect our ears is to neglect our soul.

TRUSTING OUR EARS

It is estimated that the ear is about ten times more accurate in its perceptions than the eye. For instance, there is nothing comparable to an "optical illusion" in the auditory realm. Experiments have also shown that no other sense organ can register impulses as minimal as those perceived by the ear. Furthermore, the ear can register sounds across a huge dynamic range, far greater than that which the eye can perceive without damage.[3] The ratio of intensity between the faintest and loudest sound the human ear can hear is one trillion to one.

Hans Kayser, a German scientist who developed a theory of harmonics in the 1920s based on the law of Lambdoma*, explains that the

* The law of Lambdoma is a series of numbers and mathematical proportions that enables us to understand how harmony in music follows a ratio system of whole numbers. Also see golden mean (chapter fourteen).

ear is the only human sense organ able to perceive both numerical quantity and numerical value. For instance, not only can the ear recognize numerical proportions in music, as in the octave 1:2 or the fifth 2:3, but at the same time it can hear values that it perceives as specific notes: C, G, F, and so on. (Nonmusicians will understand the ratios of musical intervals when we approach the study of Nada Yoga in chapter ten.) In other words, the element of sensing (the tone) is fused with the element of thinking (the numerical proportion). The ear is the only organ capable of doing this with remarkable precision. This is why, as Joachim-Ernst Berendt explains, "even an unmusical person can hear whether an octave is correct or not, because his ear can actually measure whether the higher tone really swings with a frequency twice that of the lower one. But nobody can see that a color emits a light frequency twice that of another one."[4] My point here is that the ears have amazing accuracy and unitive powers; "they can translate mathematical quantities into sense perceptions, conscious experiences into subconscious impressions, measurable things into immeasurable ones, abstract concepts into matters of soul, and vice versa." This unique capability allows the ears to function as a gateway to the soul.

THE EAR AS GATEWAY TO THE SOUL

By not paying enough attention to the sonic aspect of situations, we are neglecting the feminine counterpart of our visual experiences. Sound is powerfully linked to our feelings; it causes our cells and tissues to vibrate, activating a range of experience far beyond what the eyes are capable of perceiving by themselves. Obviously, we need both hearing and vision to feel complete and to protect ourselves, yet too frequently we ignore the information that comes to us through our ears and registers in our soul. There is a level of truth in this information that we have not learned to address, perhaps because of the deep introspection that it requires, and certainly because we do not trust this sense organ sufficiently. Imagine your boss or coworker saying something to you, and you replying: "I hear you, but there is an emotion underneath your words that indicates something else. Can we talk about that?"

Here is a simple experiment to demonstrate the ear's power. First, turn off the sound on your television and notice how your awareness is drawn out of your body and into the television screen. Next, turn on the sound, cover your eyes with both palms, and just listen to the program. Notice how your awareness deepens and how strongly you are drawn *into* your body. Finally, open your eyes and observe how much life, energy, and meaning the sound brings to the visual. You will also notice how, when vision and sound are partnered, your body awareness is drawn more strongly into your visual encounters — a stark contrast to the no-sound visuals you first experienced. Vision is an awesome capacity, but we need to become more conscious of how our culture neglects the ears in favor of the eyes — and what's at stake when we allow this to happen.

Joachim-Ernst Berendt cautions that people who live mainly through their eyes lead not only a diminished spiritual life, but also a less "precise" life than those more attuned to their hearing. We do not realize it sufficiently, but helping our children develop their hearing skills will guide them more safely through life's challenges. Better hearing increases self-awareness. Our eyes, if not complemented with effective listening skills, can easily deceive us.

Psychologists often remark that one of the most common complaints in counseling is that the other person is not listening. As sound yogis, we learn to listen not just with the mind but also with the whole body. This complete listening allows for bidirectional communication, which is vital if we want to function powerfully as a team, whether within our family, among our friends, with professional colleagues, or in an educational setting. This wholesome attunement replicates the optimal function of any living organism, whose cells share information through resonance. Molecular biologist Candice Pert, in her groundbreaking work *Molecules of Emotions,*[5] explains that hormones and neurotransmitters throughout the human organism communicate with each other through distinctive vibrational sympathies. In other words, when there is harmony in the body, our cells are humming along with an empathic music that minimizes dissonance. To fall out of tune is to break down communication among our cells and to literally lose the music. The same applies in our businesses, schools, governments, and families.

Sound is closely associated with the soul — the part of us that reflects something deep and eternal. This is why most illnesses indicate soul issues, and why therefore both sound and music — the language of our soul — can help restore our health. As mentioned, many ancient cultures viewed physical illness as a lack of harmony in the body; they used sound and music to restore this natural condition. A "sound body" literally produces harmonious music. Western health practitioners are beginning to realize the role of sound and music in the healing process as exploration, discoveries, and miracles in music therapies continue to gather force.[6]

ACHIEVING BALANCE

Women have always been closer to their bodies than men due to hormonal processes that are rhythmically attuned to nature. I believe that the biological capability to nourish a child in the womb and birth it into the world renders women naturally more comfortable with their bodies and their sexuality than men. Feminine qualities such as love, endurance, compassion, intimate wisdom of the body, and the capacity to nurture, birth, and connect deeply with others can be reinstated in our lives and our society by developing our ears. Sadly, modern life has forced many women to allow the masculine in them to dominate, greatly depriving Western culture of the nurturing power of the feminine. The fact that outward physical appearance dominates our appreciation of true beauty — and often prevents us from discovering the deeper essence of a person — is another indication of the value we place on the eye over the ear.

Reinstating hearing to its proper role will change both the way our culture relates to women and the way men and women relate to the feminine within themselves and in each other. This is important for our culture, our species, and the planet as a whole, but it has to start with each of us as individuals. Let us not hold back out of fear that developing the ear and its feminine power will engender vulnerability or weakness. What you will discover with the Yoga of Sound is that the ego, which is usually fortified by eye-based knowledge and judgment, is actually the most fearful and vulnerable part of ourselves, especially when estranged from the soul. The soul, on the other hand, which is developed through spiritual practice, is strong and fearless. Through practicing the Yoga of Sound, the ego and soul can function as a composite whole, complementing each other and working together to derive the deepest level of meaning and fulfillment from life.

The Upanishads, an ancient Hindu scripture, teaches that the soul can be our friend or our enemy. This is the great tension we all face and struggle with daily. Yoga is a process that brings together these opposite yet complementary aspects of our being: the individual and the cosmic, masculine and feminine, rational and intuitive, ego and soul. Developing "soul force" is as important as developing a healthy ego.

SOUND AND FORM

OUR EXPERIMENT with the television illustrates how fundamental sound is to the reality of our existence. Sound manifests in the form of waves, as do many other phenomena including light. Although our auditory range prevents us from hearing all of these frequencies as tones, at some level of our being we sense and are affected by these waves. Where the body leaves off, the mind begins; where the mind ends, soul begins, and soul merges into spirit at some level because it comes from spirit — from the image and likeness of the Divine in which it was created. I like to think that our ears actually extend into our mind, the soul, and realms of spirit in ways that make us receptive to all the waveforms of our universe. This is the perspective that guides the vision of the sound yogi. "Touch a stone and move a star," said William Blake.

The speculation that sound might be a wave phenomenon grew out of observations of water waves by early Greek philosophers such as Chrysippus (c. 240 B.C.) and Aristotle (384–322 B.C.). A wave is described as an oscillatory disturbance that moves away from a source and transports matter over large distances.[7] This is why our use of sound can actually affect the rest of the universe or affect our own body, which is also characterized by vibratory phenomena.

In the early years of the last century, Swiss scientist Hans Jenny founded a field of study called "cymatics," derived from the Greek word *kyma,* meaning "wave."[8] Cymatics visually demonstrates the relationship between sound and form — a relationship intuited by early Greek philosophers. "A stone," said Plato, "is frozen music." Jeff Volk, a poet, video artist, and publisher who promotes the study of cymatics, explains that for fourteen years Jenny conducted experiments in which he animated inert powders, pastes, and liquids into lifelike, flowing forms that mirrored patterns found throughout nature, art, and architecture. All these patterns were created using simple sine-wave vibrations (pure tones) within the human auditory range. Ancient Buddhists understood that "form is emptiness." In other words, all the forms we perceive are really vibrations arising out of a void and then disappearing back into it, a statement corroborated by modern physics.

Put simply, sound is infused with intelligence — an organizing principle that shapes the forms we perceive through our eyes. Many of the common natural patterns we see around us are a physical representation of vibration, or the way sound manifests into form. Biologist Rupert Sheldrake, in his groundbreaking work *A New Science of Life* (which was written at the ashram where I lived), refers to these organizing principles as "morphogenetic fields" — blueprints that organize matter and energy into their final intended forms. Thus, a cat embryo develops into a cat and a mango seed grows into a mango tree.[9]

In our bodies, DNA helps regenerate our cells and enables them to develop into healthy units. Without proper nutrition, explains Dr. Dharma Singh Khalsa (a rare combination of M.D. and yogi), DNA often becomes damaged, resulting in imperfect replication that, among other things, contributes to the process of aging. We can use primordial sounds and vibrations, along with a healthy lifestyle, to nurture our DNA, says Dr. Khalsa.[10] Mirroring Khalsa's findings, Dr. Deepak Chopra states: "Starting with DNA, the whole body unfolds into many levels, and at each one . . . the sequence of sound comes first. Therefore, putting a primordial sound back into the body is like reminding it what station it should be tuned in to."[11]

In this way, sound also configures our energy into definite emotional states. The power of a two-year-old to overtake our mental preoccupations with a single scream, the turmoil we experience in listening to the anguished groans of someone in pain, or the way the delightful gurgling of a newborn infant causes our heart to overflow with love are just a few examples that illustrate the point that *sound is energy.* It is this principle that guides the sound yogi to manipulate and use sound for higher spiritual purposes.

Of course, as I mentioned in the introduction, sound's power can also be destructive. Dorothy Retallack, an American musician, singer, and researcher, found that prolonged exposure to the note F for specific periods of time actually killed certain plants.[12] You may be aware of ultrasound products that keep pests out of our homes by negatively affecting their nervous systems. And it is no secret that ultrasonic weaponry is actively being researched by the American military, which has recently developed the loudest sound in history — ten thousand times louder than the sound of a space shuttle taking off — to detect the presence of submarines in our territorial waters. This Low Frequency Active (LFA) sonar technology is known to cause fatal brain hemorrhaging in whales and dolphins, not to mention its effects on human divers. Should this sound be deployed worldwide, as would happen in times of war, we might even destroy algae and other vital biological life-forms upon which our very existence depends.*

On September 25, 2003, I gave a benefit concert involving mantras for Seaflow, a grassroots organization that lobbies for the rights of marine wildlife. Within a few weeks, an injunction was brought against the U.S. Navy prohibiting the use of LFA technology in habitat areas and marine migratory routes. Obviously, there is coincidence in the timing, and I certainly cannot claim any credit for the injunction; all credit goes to the efforts of Seaflow. Yet this provides some indication of what the focused power of mantra chanting with intention can achieve.

Even the destructive capacity of sound can be put to productive use, as in the case of the lithotripter, a medical machine developed in Germany that can dissolve gallstones and kidney stones without surgery by bombarding them with sound waves. This capacity of sound to dissolve obstructions in our body and mind is one of the key principles on which the Yoga of Sound is based.

Sound is energy, and sound configures energy to give it form. To be yogis is to devote our lives and our capabilities toward creating and

---

* For more information on LFA sonar technology, visit www.seaflow.org.

sustaining harmony within ourselves and in our world. The Yoga of Sound shows us how we can do this as a regular practice.

THE INTUITIVE POWER OF THE EAR

The ear is the first organ to develop in the fetus and the last organ to stop functioning during the process of death. This prominence at the beginning and end of our life cycle indicates that the ear may hold valuable keys to the mysteries of life. Ancient cultures were acutely aware of this, particularly the indigenous shamans who mediated between the outer natural world and the inner dimension of spirit. While they relied on dreams and visions to provide them with insight into health conditions, sound was often their vehicle for channeling healing energy and intentions into the sick or distressed individual.

The Siberian shamans of the Tuva region have an extraordinary capacity to produce four simultaneous tones in their voices. These sonic meditations awaken a dormant force of tremendous magnitude in the listener, as evident from the audio recording *Deep in the Heart of the Tuva.*[13] In an interview with one of the performers on the album, a Siberian shaman named Ondar explained: "*Hoomei* [multitoned throat singing] is not simply singing. When you perform hoomei, that which you want to express must truly come from within your soul." Siberian shamans also use sound to drive away negative forces or spirits that afflict the person in need of healing.

While our eyes help light our path through this world, we also know that we came from darkness and will return to darkness. This darkness, which represents the inability of the analytical mind to fathom the depths of consciousness, is revealed through our explorations in Sound Yoga. As you will discover in the coming chapters, the Yoga of Sound can help us move as a species toward a life in which mystery is as important as information, depth of emotion is as important as rational thinking, and spiritual awakening is as important as worldly pleasure. Where we cannot see, sound can guide us.

> *No matter how deeply I go into myself my God is dark, and like webbing made of a hundred roots that drink in silence.*
>
> **Rainer Maria Rilke**[14]

CHAPTER 2

YOKING OURSELVES TO THE COSMIC

To understand the Yoga of Sound, we must first examine what the term "yoga" has come to mean in the West. In this chapter, we look at Hatha Yoga — the popular form of yoga postures and breathing practiced in most yoga studios — as well as samadhi, *the end goal of enlightened yogic consciousness.* Samadhi, *as we shall see, is not some esoteric ideal, but a practical and meaningful fulfillment of human potential, accessible to every one of us.*

For the past three hundred years, since the time of philosopher René Descartes and mathematician Isaac Newton, Western thinking has become increasingly entrenched in an unhealthy perception of the world as completely separate from the human mind. This Newtonian-Cartesian view of the world as a machine is now changing with the emergence of quantum physics, which views the universe as comprised of waves of energy networked in an inseparable whole, each wave affecting others in definite ways.

Yoga has come as a great gift from the East to the West because it heals the fragmentation created by a mechanistic worldview at the fundamental physical-sexual level. After hundreds of years of denigration of the body in Christian theology and prayer, Hatha Yoga allows the West to see the body with fresh eyes — as an instrument to be tuned, rather than subjugated. And as we saw in chapter one, yoga also counteracts the mechanistic stress of our world. But the goal of yoga, as it has been practiced in the East for thousands of years, is something greater: *samadhi,* an ecstatic union that encompasses all the dimensions of our being — body, soul, and spirit.

Yoga has several important definitions that come from the agrarian culture in which it was born. The word "yoga" is primarily derived from the Sanskrit root *yuj,* or *yugam,* meaning "to yoke," symbolizing the wholeness that occurs when the individual self — the ego or psyche — is joined, or yoked, with a vision of the cosmic. Today this sense of belonging to the universe is crucial to our building a global community inclusive of all life.

Yoga also embodies the agrarian image of oxen *yoked* to the plough, as the practice of yoga cultivates the ground of our being, the soil of our soul. The harvest is an abundance of spiritual experiences that bring joy and fulfillment to the deepest parts of our selves. This cultivation takes *effort,* another definition of yoga, which then translates into energy. The more energy we put into our spiritual practice, the more we receive.

Finally, yoga means *path.* The steps that constitute the way of yoga have been researched over thousands of years. The effects of yogic practice are easily verified by direct personal experience. No belief is required; just practice the steps and enjoy the benefits, which you can compare and share with others on the path. It is this pragmatic credibility that has given yoga such wide appeal, easily cutting across religious and cultural boundaries. But reaching the ultimate goal of samadhi requires following the practice to its culmination.

YOGA IN THE WEST

"YOGA" IS NOW a household term in the West. But the yoga that has become popular here is just one form of yoga: *Hatha Yoga.* The roots of Hatha Yoga can be traced back to the second century B.C., when Patanjali,* the father of classical yoga, codified it in his famous *Yoga Sutras.* This expanded form of Hatha Yoga, known as *Raja Yoga* or "the royal path," is a holistic approach that combines the systematic flow of

* Some scholars believe that the Patanjali who authored the *Yoga Sutras* was also the Patanjali who wrote a famous commentary on Sanskrit grammar: this person lived in 200 B.C. Other scholars place the Patanjali credited with the *Yoga Sutras* between 100 and 200 A.D. The problem is that the author's name, Patanjali, does not appear anywhere in the *Yoga Sutras.*

body postures, breathing practices, and mind-focusing techniques with moral and social obligations that act as a prerequisite for psycho-spiritual exercises. The form of Hatha Yoga commonly taught in most yoga studios dispenses with the moral prerequisites and relies mostly on physical postures, stretches, and a modest amount of breath control. This style of Hatha Yoga could well have emerged from the *Goraknath* lineage of yogis, a militant sect that developed in the Middle Ages.

In its fullest sense, yoga is a form of prayer through the conduit of our bodies. When I began my life as a Benedictine monk and Hindu yogi — a unique combination under the direction of Bede Griffiths — I was shocked to read stories of St. Benedict rolling in thorns and St. Francis of Assisi plunging naked into the snow. These acts were performed to eliminate sexual arousal — a rather violent reaction to natural tendencies, it seemed to me. While it might have worked for them during that period in human evolution, it is a disastrous option for us today. We might take our cue from some of the yogic Christian mystics of the Middle Ages, who had a more balanced view. St. Mechtilde of Magdeburg, a Benedictine Abbess, cautioned: "Do not disdain your body, for the soul is just as safe in its body as in the Kingdom of Heaven."[1]

While the physical fitness aspect of yoga is extremely important, we should avoid seeing it as an end in itself. We can therefore differentiate between Hatha Yoga, used to strengthen the physical body and develop the nervous system, and Raja Yoga, an eight-limbed system intended to create optimal conditions for ultimate spiritual enlightenment. The eight limbs are *yama** and *niyama,* self-restraint and religious observances, which comprise ten codes (five each) of moral and social conduct; *asana* and *pranayama,* posture and breath control; *pratyahara* and *dharana,* withdrawal from the senses and equanimity of mind; and *dhyana* and samadhi, meditation and enlightenment.

The eight limbs of Raja Yoga provide a holistic paradigm. The advanced Hatha yogi uses complex techniques of locking and moving energy through the body, a sophisticated cleansing process, and intricate muscular contractions, all of which make the body a holy temple. But

---

* The five codes of yama are *ahimsa* (not causing injury), *satya* (truthfulness), *asteya* (not stealing), *brahmacharya* (celibacy), and *aparigraha* (not coveting).

these practices still only focus on the third and fourth limbs of Raja Yoga. Hatha Yoga teachers in the West are beginning to sense the need for the larger holistic paradigm; the role of sound in yoga practice must be explored within this context. The use of mantras and meditation techniques involving sound and deep listening enable the yogi to develop the fifth, sixth, seventh, and eighth limbs of Raja Yoga. These limbs pertain directly to the enlightenment of soul and spiritual realization.

Mantras — the sounds of yoga — provide the fuel and energy for any system of yoga. Whether one practices Hatha Yoga, Karma Yoga (the path of selfless action), Gnana Yoga (the path of intellectual inquiry), or Bhakti Yoga (the path of devotion), the attunement to spiritual vibrations through music, silence, movement, or the flow of energy in the body clearly involves the underlying principles and teachings of the Yoga of Sound.

THE TRUE MEANING AND PURPOSE OF YOGA

In India, yoga has always been somewhat antireligious and antigovernmental. Yet despite its utter self-reliance and independence, and a history of refusing to submit to the status quo, it has always managed to stay focused on its highest goal: samadhi. Credit the spiritual vitality of Hinduism as a tradition, which continues to the present day. Each year, Asha and I make a pilgrimage to South India with our students. We are repeatedly struck by the intensity of Hindu devotion and how it compares to life in the West. My mentor, Bede Griffiths, once wrote that the West had banished God. We see this banishment in the sterility of our public places; reminders of the sacred appear nowhere. Because Hatha Yoga in America lacks the spiritual container it had in India, we must protect, nurture, and encourage it to grow.

The Yoga of Sound, I believe, can usher more soul into yoga as it is transplanted to the West and can help Westerners achieve the deepest fulfillment possible through their yoga practice. This is already happening through the widespread use of *kirtan,* the call-and-response chanting of the names and attributes of Hindu Gods. However, kirtan is only one avenue to the depths of sound yoga — albeit an important one, since it reaches into the heart. Kirtan is the first step toward recovering the soul of Hatha Yoga, but much more is possible when all the streams of sonic mysticism are taken into account. In chapter three, I will explain why it is imperative that other streams of Sound Yoga be included in the lifestyle of the present-day yogi.

Although yoga is not a religion and doesn't require belief in any specific deity, yoga in India has always recognized a higher power in the universe and has inspired devotion to this power, regardless of the name one might choose for it. The *Bhagavad Gita,* the great spiritual classic on yoga, expounds on the value of Karma, Bhakti, and Gnana Yoga. The *Gita,* which shows that all paths lead to the same end, reserves a special place for devotion, which is passion and love for the hidden mystery of life.

Yet despite the devotional container of Hindu spirituality, even yogis in India have been distracted from the goal of samadhi; they become preoccupied with the acquisition of paranormal powers, known as *siddhis,* or enamored with austerities that express extreme indifference to suffering. This has often led to criticism of yoga, especially among Western Christians. The Buddha, who was strongly influenced by yogic discipline, remedied this indifference to the suffering of others (those less tempered in the spiritual life as well as those who are mentally deluded) through the central ideal of the *bodhisattva,* who refuses ultimate enlightenment until all sentient beings have attained it. The bodhisattva also vows to do everything he or she can, both personally and socially, to assist in the process. This Buddhist attitude of the ultimate elimination of suffering is well worth including in a postmodern approach to yoga; as we move into a global culture and society, yogis must desire samadhi for all humanity. The Buddha also proposed a middle way between the extremities of austerity and indulgence — a vision that fits well with that of yogic harmony taught in the *Gita.*

ECSTATIC UNION: THE GOAL OF YOGA

Within the term Hatha Yoga, the syllable "ha" refers to the sun and "tha" to the moon, suggesting two opposite yet complementary energies that manifest in the body and the world. We perceive these distinctive energetic qualities in many forms: in gender, through masculine and feminine; in electromagnetic attraction, through positive and negative poles; and in centripetal and centrifugal forces, which pull toward or away from a central axis. Through the practice of Hatha Yoga, these energies must be fused together to produce the union of samadhi.

Samadhi is an ecstatic form of enlightenment. It is also progressive, moving beyond the initial ecstasy experienced on the physical level to deeper and more expansive states of consciousness. Millions of yogis throughout India who have dedicated their lives to yoga, generation after generation for thousands of years, bear witness to the fact that this spiritual ecstasy is far more than what the world can offer.

Yet there is only one enlightenment. Christian and Buddhist monks, Native American shamans, Sufi dervishes, and Jewish Hasidim all share the mystical realm, involving similar experiences. They attest to the same ecstatic, blissful states of consciousness. What we can explore, regardless of our religious persuasion, is how yoga — through both its sonic and physical routines — can enhance our spiritual life and motivate our spiritual practice to its most sublime possibilities. This practice will not interfere with any of our religious commitments; it does not, for instance, require us to give up faith in Jesus Christ. Yoga should, in fact, enhance our experience of the mystery of Christ and help us recover our mystical depth.

Samadhi, at its deepest level, is our natural state of grace. This same ecstasy is funneled through all our activities whenever we are truly at one with what we are doing. Yet the fullness of samadhi often escapes our grasp because many of our activities have misdirected agendas or seek a limited good. The use of mantra keeps us attuned to the high vibration of samadhi and moves our activities toward that goal. We have glimpses of samadhi through many of our activities and experiences, but the fullness of this experience lies in a profound surrender of self. Sports players often speak of "the zone" — a mental, physical, and emotional state in which they are one with their play. As Tom Cruise advised Cuba Gooding, Jr., in the film *Jerry McGuire,* "You've got to play for the sake of the game, not for the money or what your sponsor could do for you." When we put this principle into practice, "yoga happens." But such surrender does not come easily to us. Once again, mantra provides us with a way to surrender our anxieties, fears, and the egoic pride that sometimes interferes with the ecstatic flow of consciousness in our body.

Samadhi may not come easily to all of us, but this does not mean that it is far removed or inaccessible to a normal human being living in the world. It is not an esoteric illusion. It is our natural state of consciousness — a state that lies hidden under the camouflage of mental activity, a state that is forgotten because of our excessive preoccupation with this world.

Hinduism teaches that we are in this body to work through those habits and patterns that have become encrusted and that prevent our soul from expanding. Expansion is the true nature of the soul. Like the universe, the soul must constantly expand or suffer from a psychic claustrophobia that will eventually eat us up from the inside. Then, like a black hole, we will consume light instead of radiating it. The soul, too, can shrink into a confined space prescribed by the ego and its limited vision; like a genie trapped in a bottle, it becomes impotent until it is released from its confinement.

The Yoga of Sound, through the use of mantras, helps release the soul from the spell that binds it to a hardened ego. In the end it offers *moksha* — liberation from self-induced suffering — which then opens the door to samadhi. Suffering, in the Hindu tradition, is the result of ignorance, and yoga is a way out of this ignorance.

Building our spiritual life is like building a house. In helping develop the limbic, nervous, and circulatory systems of our physical body, Hatha Yoga is akin to having a strong foundation and structure. But building a great house does not satisfy us unless we invite our family and friends to share it with us and celebrate life within its walls. While focusing mostly on the house itself, Hatha Yoga in the West seems to have forgotten the life that must dwell inside it. Spirit and Divinity must be consciously invited into this home, this temple, and that is where the Yoga of Sound can play an important and necessary role.

Although the ecstasy of samadhi is present in all our activities, the fullness of samadhi doesn't come cheap. Authentic samadhi involves the whole person and every aspect of being; this is why we must learn to view yoga in its broadest sense. The expansive union of samadhi encompasses everything — all levels of being, all states of consciousness, from the microscopic to the macroscopic, from the energy of photons, electrons, cells, and molecules to our energetic empathy with complex organisms and great stellar bodies. Mantras establish this union to form dynamic energy relationships between our soul and the rest of the universe, resulting in a bidirectional flow of intelligence that enriches our consciousness and creates the ecstasy that is samadhi.

CHAPTER 3

THE MARRIAGE OF BODY AND SOUL

In this chapter, we will examine how the Yoga of Sound, through the practice of mantra, fits into the larger historical context of the Hindu tradition, and I will introduce the four distinct streams of sacred sound as yoga.

The Yoga of Sound, together with *Ayurveda* (the Indian tradition of healing) and Hatha Yoga, emerges from the ancient Indian cultural and spiritual vortex of the *Rishis.* The Rishis were visionary seers and poets, like the ancient Celtic bards, who were attuned to the vibratory structures of the universe. They were also the authors of the *Vedas,* the most ancient of Hindu scriptures. The spiritual visions of the Rishis during meditation and yoga practice were so profound that their visions translated into sounds, which were then encoded in mystic formulas called mantras. Mantras, as sonic structures of energy and consciousness, form the basis of the Yoga of Sound in the same way that postures or positions (asanas) form the basis of Hatha Yoga practice.

Broadly speaking, as Hinduism evolved, the Yoga of Sound developed as a science of consciousness, Ayurveda as a science of healing, Hatha Yoga as a science of physical strength and balance, and Raja Yoga — the eight-limbed expansion of Hatha Yoga — as a holistic science of the body, mind, and spirit. Similarly, *Tantra* developed as the science of energy, and *Vaastu* as the science of architecture — the Indian counterpart of Chinese Feng Shui.

The key difference between Hatha Yoga and Sound Yoga is that, while Hatha Yoga primarily develops the infrastructure of the physical body and its nervous system, the Yoga of Sound works essentially with the transformation, restoration, and reconstitution of the energies of the soul through channels known as *nadis* (from the same root as *nada*), which are subtle channels of the chakra system related to the soul's infrastructure. While Hatha Yoga optimizes the performance of physical organs such as the heart and the lungs, the Yoga of Sound optimizes the performance of energy vortexes known as chakras, which govern our emotional, psychic, and spiritual states of consciousness. Whereas Hatha Yoga teaches us how to effectively manage and purify the dense aspects of our being (blood, cells, and tissue), the Yoga of Sound maintains the subtler aspects of our being (thoughts, emotions, and states of consciousness) and helps keep them free of psychic and spiritual toxicity.

As Indian culture and spirituality evolved, these branches of study became specialized approaches of their own, but they continued to draw from a common pool of spiritual wisdom and consciousness. The Yoga of Sound developed its specialty around the principles of *mantra shastra* and *mantra vidya,* which are the rules and knowledge governing mantras, together with the rituals and ceremonies conducted around the use of sacred sound.

THE FOUR STREAMS OF SONIC MYSTICISM

THE SOPHISTICATION of the ancient Hindu mind is evident in their six major schools of philosophy, the complexity of their five-thousand-year-old cities, and their astounding mathematical capabilities, which include the origination of our modern number system — a discovery no less important than the mastery of fire, the development of agriculture, or the invention of the wheel.[1] What differentiates the Hindu brilliance in logic and rational thought from its Hellenistic parallel is that Hindus were very aware of the intellect's limitations. They understood that only the feminine intuitive mind was capable of grasping the deepest spiritual truths in powerful flashes of intuition. The Rishis were expert at this process, and they left behind a gargantuan legacy of mantras to help awaken the same flashes of intuitive perception in us. This huge body of sacred sound is essentially encoded in the most ancient of Hindu scriptures, collectively known as the *Vedas,* which date to between 1500 and 500 B.C. The mantras of the Vedas were originally an oral tradition that was refined over many millennia.

While the Vedas form the first formalized stream of Sound Yoga, there are actually four streams of sonic mysticism that characterize the Hindu tradition. Although each stream is distinct, they are interrelated. For purposes of functionality and effectiveness, I have attributed relevant yogic terms to each of these streams: Shabda Yoga is the use of sacred sound derived from the Vedic tradition of mantra; Shakti Yoga is the sonic aspect of the Tantric tradition; and Bhava Yoga represents the devotional chanting of the Bhakti tradition. Nada Yoga, the classical term for Sound Yoga that has become popular in the West in recent years, is insufficient to cover the breadth and depth of sonic applications in yoga practice, as I will explain; I therefore treat it as a fourth stream. In addition to the introductory material in this chapter, we will explore each stream in detail in part three.

The Yoga of Sound brings together all four of these streams in a comprehensive approach, allowing them to inform and support one another in a single system. Each of these four paths is normally learned in a separate school under experts who are usually proficient in only one of them. For the express purpose of providing the postmodern yogi with a balanced and wholesome sonic spirituality, I have brought together the essential and most useful aspects of each of these four paths in a cross-disciplinary system. I feel that we need such a unified system in order to have a deeply fulfilled life in the present world.

Shabda Yoga (Vedic Mantras): Architecture of the Gods and Keys to Intuitive Knowledge

***VED* MEANS** "to know" — not to know about, but a knowing that is direct, intimate, wholesome, and multidimensional. Vedic mantras, which we will study under the broad stream of Shabda Yoga, combine sound, word, and meaning to generate flashes of intuition, spiritual perception, and poetic inspiration.

The Yoga of Sound has accompanied the practice of Hatha Yoga postures since Hinduism's earliest beginnings. During the Vedic age, and probably long before, practitioners of yoga remained in a yogic posture (asana) for a long time in order to invoke a particular deity and develop specific yogic powers. To achieve these powers, specific mantras were partnered with the postures; the lotus posture *(padmasana)* and the tree *(vrikshasana)* were common asanas used to obtain *mantra siddhi,* or powers associated with mantras. Toward the end of the Vedic age (500 B.C.), during the period of the great Indian epics,* we know that mantras invoking Shiva, Vishnu, or Brahma — the three principal deities of Hinduism that evolved out of the Vedic age — were coupled with asanas. Prior to this, it is likely that many obscure and secret Tantric mantras were used to develop yogic powers.

According to ancient Hindu cosmology, the Divine maintains harmony and balance in the universe and protects the various parts of the universe through self-emanating powers known as *vibhutis.* In the Vedic tradition, these governing powers are celebrated as the *devas,* or "shining ones," much like the angels of the Bible. To live harmoniously with these unseen powers was considered essential for the well-being of the community, a perspective common to all ancient cultures. In Hinduism, mantras were associated with these cosmic powers and regarded as a sort of code that could link human consciousness to specific emanations of Divine power, just as the name of Jesus can connect us to his holy presence and power. Effective use of the mantras could therefore introduce in our own bodies and minds the same balance, harmony, and protection that was prevalent in the universe.

For the yogis of the Vedic age, the use of mantras helped maintain *rta* — pronounced "ruh-thah" — the sense of cosmic order and harmony that the Rishis perceived as prevailing throughout the universe. The notion that sonic consonance and harmony dominated the cosmos was shared by all ancient cultures, including the early Greek philosophers. Later, in the seventeenth century, Johannes Kepler mathematically proved this concept through his Third Law of Planetary Motion, which showed that a great number of musical harmonies exist among the angular velocities of the planets in relationship to the sun. Musicologist Joachim-Ernst Berendt explains: "Not only the planetary

* The great Indian epics, the *Mahabharata* and the *Ramayana,* are comparable to the *Iliad* and the *Odyssey.* The *Bhagavad Gita* appears in the *Mahabharata.* The *Ramayana* tells the story of Rama.

orbits, but also the proportions within these orbits follow the laws of harmonics, much more than statistical probability would lead us to expect. Out of the seventy-eight tones created by the different planetary proportions, seventy-four belong to the major scale (a most harmonic sequence) — a truly overwhelming configuration that no 'chance' in the world will be able to explain."[2]

The uniqueness of Vedic mantras lies in their cosmic resonance, which can be viewed as an architecture of the Gods, corresponding to our solar systems and galaxies, which are the great temples of our universe. Vedic mantras embody a human replica of this cosmic architecture, providing a sense of protection to the user by building a palpable force-field around the soul. This protective force-field becomes a means by which we can align ourselves with the harmony of the universe and generate harmony in our own lives and relationships.

In Vedic brahminism,* the whole was viewed as being greater than its parts, the sum total of which could be glimpsed in flashes of powerful intuition. Grammar and phonetics played an important role in the awakening of this intuition, as the process came to rely on the structure of the sentence. Proper syntax, poetic nuance, and the spiritual power of individual words were combined into the use of language as the means toward yogic union and enlightenment. The entire sentence and the flow of sentences, one into another, were a type of *vinyasa*. Vinyasa, for Hatha yoga practitioners, is an arrangement of postures that flow into one another to offer a complete yoga workout of all the parts and muscles of the body. In the Vedic world, words were like yoga postures, used to awaken spiritual illumination; the knowledge of Sanskrit grammar helped one understand the spiritual and energetic relationship among individual words.

In the Vedic approach, mantras were also viewed as vehicles of the spirit realm, as they transported both the chanter and the listener to specific states of consciousness. The rhythmic and poetic meters of the Vedas were therefore compared to horses, their counterparts in the material world that help us travel physical distances.

* Vedic brahminism was the formal institution of the Vedic world. Brahmins were the priestly caste who oversaw the procedures of rituals and mantras, similar to the Levites of the Hebrew world.

Shakti Yoga (Tantric Mantras): Alphabets of Divine Energy

SHAKTI YOGA,* another stream of Sound Yoga that we will study, comes from Tantrism. *Tantra* means "fabric," and it describes the universe as an intermeshing web of energetic relationships — a view that is identical to current discoveries in particle physics, cited in chapter two. According to Tantric cosmology, the individual letters of the Sanskrit language, from which mantras are constructed, are derived from sonic structures that form the basic building blocks of the universe. Here we see the reverse of the Vedic view of language; in this case, the part — the individual letter — is greater than the whole. Hence, in Tantric philosophy, every part of the human body, including the genitals and excretory organs, is sacred — just as every part of the earth's body is held as sacred.

Tantra has become popular in the West because of its strong association with sexuality, in the same way that Hatha Yoga has gained popularity because of its amazing fitness routines. A key difference between the Vedic and Tantric uses of mantras is that, in Tantrism, the part is viewed as being greater than the whole because it contains the whole. This perspective, too, is corroborated by modern scientific discoveries such as the hologram, in which the whole is indeed present in every part, even when the part is broken up into little pieces. Another illustration of this principle comes from a controlled biological experiment, in which worms kept in a dark box were shocked with electricity when flashed with a bright light. Later, these worms were ground up and fed to a second batch of worms that were not put through the same shock treatment — yet they, too, reacted by coiling up in response to the flashed light in exactly the same way as the first set.[3]

Tantra functions on the principle that energy is constantly being exchanged among all the parts of the universe through an intricate system of channels. The human body is viewed as a microcosm of the universe, replicating this complex network of universal energy channels. The sounds of the individual Sanskrit letters and the basic

* Although the Tantric tradition is older than the Vedic, formal Tantric texts only started to appear around 500 A.D. Tantric influence is evident in many aspects of the Vedic tradition, especially in South India.

sounds of human energy, such as grunts, groans, and other inarticulate sounds, are codified in mantras that represent the flow and control of energy in and through the human organism. These basic sound structures, also known as *bijas* ("seed syllables"), are extracted from fundamental sound forms that make up the energy of the universe.

While Hatha Yoga postures help align and strengthen the body's complex network of energy channels, in Tantrism the mantric sounds employed by the yogi wield the energetic force *(kundalini)*, awaken siddhi (spiritual powers and perceptions), and lead to the realization of ecstatic union that is both sexual and spiritual. In Tantrism, the use of sacred sound therefore becomes important in the way we relate to our sexuality and the flow of energy in and through our body. Through the use of yoga and sacred sound, Tantrism teaches us to respect our sexuality and to connect more intimately with the innate intelligence of the body. Imagine such a teaching as a part of the high school curriculum, helping our teens effectively manage and channel their sexual energy, then carry this ability into adulthood and eventually marriage.

Bhava Yoga (Devotional Mantras): The Sound of Love and Sacred Relationships

Devotion is an act of relating to the Divine with love and reverence. It requires keeping the channels open in all our relationships so that the movement of energy is bidirectional, flowing from us toward the Divine and from the Divine toward us. Devotion brings us to the next stream of the Yoga of Sound tradition: Bhava Yoga, which comes to us through the Bhakti movement that is comprised of devotional sects within Hinduism. Prior to the emergence of the Bhakti movement, which spread widely in India during the Middle Ages, the common person was caught between two extremes: the institutional Vedic tradition, which relied on the precise use of ritual, posture, and sound; and the wild, untamed, eccentric Tantric tradition, which many ordinary people found strange and frightening. The former was aligned with the state, while the latter claimed self-realized spiritual authority.

Yogis have always known that devotion drives yoga practice to its depths — to the very nature of the soul. The fifth niyama* pertaining to the second limb of Raja Yoga is *Isvarapranidhana* — to lay all one's actions at the feet of God. Devotional yoga began in the pre-Christian era and developed mostly in small cults, finding its first strength in the *Alvars,* musician saints in the seventh century A.D. who hailed from my native state of Tamil Nadu. The Bhakti movement, a focused stream of devotional yoga that started around 700 A.D., gathered strength around 1300 A.D. and spread throughout India well into the seventeenth century, influencing Islam through the Sufis and inspiring the Sikhs, an Indian religious sect that developed in the sixteenth century. Musician saints began singing of the liberating power of devotional chanting and encouraged the average citizen to take up the repetition of the holy name of God. These musician and poet saints — such as Kabir, Mirabai, Tukaram, and Maanickavaachakar — sang beautiful songs that opened the heart and engendered a flowering of spiritual consciousness in the devotees. And the sounds that poured forth from these extremely accessible musician saints captured many hearts. Here, at last, was a way to find spiritual ecstasy, readily available to all without barriers of caste (another requirement of the Vedic tradition for the study of sacred sound) or the practice of austerities and countercultural behavior expected of the Tantric schools.

The bhaktas, both men and women yogis, saw themselves as feminine in relation to the Deity. Just as the Vedic mantras brought about the desired result through their precision, the bhaktas believed that the love they offered to the Divine attracted, in return, the love they sought. The bhakta also believed that one could find liberation through Divine grace, by which means the karmic process — negative energy implicit in negative actions — could be modified. In other words, devotional mantras reestablish one's relationship with the Divine, transforming past transgressions into a positive force and preventing future misdeeds.

As mentioned in the footnote on page 28, although the Tantric tradition is the oldest stream within Hinduism, it did not truly develop

* The five codes of the niyamas are *Saucha* (internal and external purity), *Santosha* (contentment), *Tapas* (austerity), *Svadhyaya* (study of religious literature and the repetition of mantras), and *Isvarapranidhana* (self-surrender to God and worship of the Divine presence).

into a formal path until around 500 A.D.; the Vedic tradition was formalized and institutionalized first, which is why it is placed first in our learning sequence. There is also a functional purpose for this sequence, which will become clear in part three, "Tradition." But from an evolutionary perspective, we can now perceive the development of sacred sound in Hinduism, from the primal sounds of sexuality and magical incantations developed in ancient Tantra, to the sculpted, refined language of Sanskrit mantras during the Vedic age, to the breakthrough in freedom from technique and the liberty of musical expression within the Bhakti movement of the Middle Ages. Here, sound touches the depths of the heart and reaches to the bottom of the soul.

These three streams also form an inward progression. Vedic mantras, which establish the expansive connections between individual consciousness and the rest of the universe, are brought home to the locus of the physical body through Tantric mantras. Both macrocosm (Shabda) and microcosm (Shakti) are then transformed in the crucible of the heart through the practice of devotion (Bhava and Bhakti). All three streams of sonic mysticism are necessary for this complete and wholesome transformation of self and the world. I often tell my students that if the world were a place of heart, devotional mantras alone would be more than sufficient to nourish our souls. But we all know that the world is not such a place, and we need to be well equipped on the soul level to take on the challenge of living with and through the powerful changes that we experience on all levels of consciousness daily.

Nada Yoga: The Science of Vibration

SHABDA, SHAKTI, and Bhava are like three sides of an equilateral triangle that symbolize the three levels of consciousness: physical, psychic/psychological, and spiritual. All three, like the three dynamic forces of Ayurveda known as *doshas*,* must be kept in balance in order to maintain optimal health and equilibrium. Nada Yoga is like a circle that passes through the three apexes of this triangle, encircling them all in its scope of sound, music, and meditation.

---

* *Dosha* means "that which changes." In Ayurvedic philosophy, the five elements — earth, water, fire, air, and space — combine in pairs to form three dynamic forces called doshas, which interact with each other.

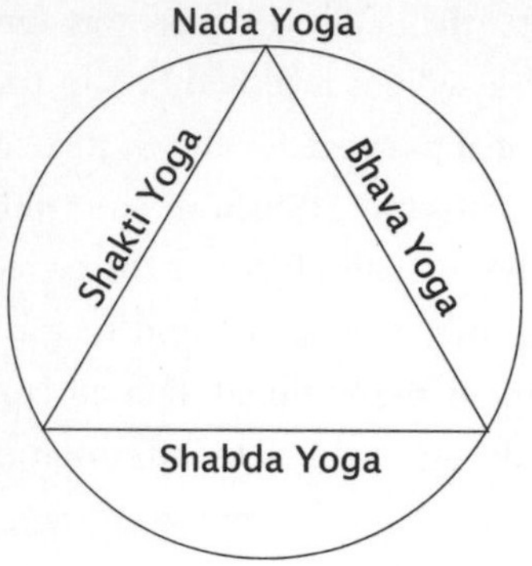

To derive maximum benefit from the other three streams of Sound Yoga, knowledge of Nada Yoga is essential. "Nada" means "sound, stream, and rushing." It is the classical term for the Yoga of Sound, and it developed alongside Hatha Yoga. Nada Yoga involves many of the postures and techniques of Hatha Yoga, but it uses them to listen deeply to the body and, through the body, to perceive hidden structures of the universe in their sonic shapes and forms.

Nada Yoga does not truly specialize in mantra, but it addresses the intervals of sound that are utilized both in music and mantra recitation. The sophistication of Nada Yoga is evident from the amazing traditions of Indian music that derive their cosmology, spirituality, and musicology from yogic consciousness. There are two such traditions: the ancient Carnatic music of the south (the tradition I was schooled in) and the Persian-influenced Hindustani music of the north. Nada Yoga provides the mantra user with both musical knowledge and meditation tools. Its rich understanding of *ragas* (musical modes that are used at specific times of the day and night to facilitate healing, harmony, and yoga), as well as its methods of deep listening to specific sounds and to silence itself, contribute significantly to the application of mantras in yoga practice. Conversely, the mantras add power and texture to both music and meditation.

In our approach to the Yoga of Sound, we will treat Nada Yoga as a fourth stream of sacred sound — one that deals with meditation, music, and deep listening. In actuality, Nada Yoga is like a great river that merges the streams of Vedic, Tantric, and devotional sound, and carries them toward the vast ocean of consciousness.

PART 2

MANTRA

THE SOUL OF YOGA

The mantra is dynamic, powerful; it will sink deeper into your consciousness . . . because the mantra is the living symbol of the Divine. As it penetrates the deeper levels of consciousness it comes to stand for the highest we can conceive of, the highest we can aspire to, the highest we can love.

Eknath Easwaran[1]

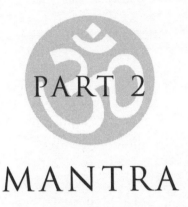

CHAPTER 4

MANTRA IN AN INTERSPIRITUAL AGE

Mantras are fascinating tools in our spiritual evolution. They constitute a language of the spiritual realm — a means of communicating with the Gods. Yet, despite their attraction, mantras also raise concerns, in part because they are difficult to understand and because they developed in one particular religious context. Mantras encompass an enormous quantity of data, and they display a great variety of applications. My objective in this chapter is to anticipate some of the common reservations about mantras and remove any mental or emotional blocks that stand in the way of our using these amazing tools of the spiritual life.

The monumental pantheon of the Gods and Goddesses in Hinduism is a collection of the tradition's most visible symbols. Many Westerners are familiar with the three main deities of Hinduism: Brahma the creator, Vishnu the preserver, and Shiva, who destroys old forms so that new ones can develop. Others may know of Ganesha, the elephant-headed son of Shiva, who removes obstacles. Saraswati, Brahma's consort and the goddess of wisdom and learning, may also be familiar. To put mantra in its proper context, people who were raised in monotheistic traditions must come to understand more of Hinduism's core philosophy. This will aid recognition of the fact that the long-perceived differences between the one God of Christianity, Islam, and Judaism and the many Gods of Hinduism is not as real as we thought.

The first Axial period — the centuries between 800 and 600 B.C., named by writer and philosopher Aldous Huxley — spawned the world's great religions. Before this time, people worshipped many primitive Gods and Goddesses, such as Baal, a Canaanite fertility deity, or the Satyrs, ancient Greek deities in the form of animals. During the first Axial period, there were several watershed occurrences: the Hebrew tradition claimed access to a supreme being known as Yahweh; Lao-tzu developed the Tao in China; Zarathustra revealed Ahura Mazda to the five-thousand-year-old Avesta religion of Iran; and the Buddha broke through to *nirvana*. During the first Axial period, the great religions were young; in their early development, they needed to be protected from misinterpretation, oppression, and external influences. Consequently, the religions developed clear guidelines about what was acceptable to their Supreme Being and what was not. Strict religious observances and discrimination of what practices were considered to be outside the faith, or dogma, helped define each religion.

The problem, especially with the Semitic traditions, was that it became the One Supreme Being *versus* the many Gods and Goddesses. The Supreme Being — Yahweh, Allah, or God the Father in Christianity — each claimed to be the one true God; all others were false, or lesser in power. The commandment "You shall not have false Gods before me" in Judaism, or the banning of graven images in Islam, both reflect this exclusivist mentality.

Regretfully, as religions developed they continued to project judgment and anger, even upon the Supreme Being they had discovered, as shown in the Koran, the Psalms, and the Old Testament. As time went on, people came to idolize or become fixated on the Supreme Being. They failed to see the value of our universe's great diversity, instead developing prejudice and exclusivity in their newfound love. Jesus' radical teachings attempted to rectify this by showing that the love of one's neighbor is as important as our love for the Divine.

Fortunately, Hinduism never fell victim to this damaging exclusivism. Like the Celtic tradition, it maintained an awareness of "pan-en-theism," meaning "everything in God." Although this idea is often misunderstood or misinterpreted, Hindus remain aware that the One is present in the many, and the many in the One. Their great tolerance and acceptance of other faiths stems from this basic understanding that the One can be accessed through any Divine manifestation because they are all emanations from the same Supreme source.

Today we have arrived at the second Axial period, a time when we recognize the perennial philosophy that underlies all religion. Many spiritually minded people acknowledge the existence of only One Supreme Being, albeit known by many names and perceived through many forms. This commingling of the One Supreme Being and the many Gods and Goddesses creates tension, as it did during the first Axial period over two thousand years ago. In the midst of this turmoil, we are all challenged to stay connected to our source in the Divine, to love our neighbor as ourselves, and to place ourselves in harmony with the energy and intelligence that surround us.

THE INTERSPIRITUAL AGE

TODAY, MANY PEOPLE believe that a single tradition cannot hold all the answers to the deep questions pressing upon us. As we evolve, we realize that our spiritual needs vary during different phases in our lives; these needs are often met by solutions from another spiritual tradition or branch of study. Sometimes psychology is more important than spiritual practice; at other times philosophy may provide more insight than psychology; and sometimes common sense rules over all. Our global community has officially entered the Interspiritual Age.

Wayne Teasdale, in his remarkable book *The Mystic Heart,* brings to our attention this beautiful term "interspirituality."[2] More and more people, he says, are being drawn to the interspiritual way, which is a simultaneous combination of paths. This does not mean that they aren't committed to any single tradition. On the contrary, they are deeply committed to *more* than one tradition. Buddhist-Jews, Hindu-Christians, and Buddhist-Christians are common hybrids. Others blend a more involved assortment, combining three or four paths. For the first time in history, we actually feel safe to openly bear witness to our spiritual preferences.

Furthermore, in the United States we have Baptists, Methodists, Seventh-Day Adventists, Catholics, Episcopalians, Presbyterians, Lutherans, Calvinists, and numerous other denominations within Christianity alone. Matthew Fox once remarked, "The present generation neither knows the difference between these denominations, nor cares about them." As we forge the structures of interspirituality, we must consider our youth and our children. Many parents, in their rejection of the idiosyncrasies and frustrations of a particular tradition, raise their children without any spiritual form whatsoever. We should feel free to explore and expose our children to all kinds of traditions, showing them the value of many perspectives and the underlying truths behind them all.

It is important that we study the Yoga of Sound and explore the power of mantra in this spirit of interspirituality and acceptance. I believe that the Yoga of Sound cuts across many boundaries. Because of its musical associations, it can transport the soul through a vast scope of possibilities, from aggressive mantra rap to sublime poetic enunciation, from raw tones to sophisticated musical phrases, from breath and dance to mathematics and cosmology. We can feel free to incorporate mantra into our own traditions, no matter what they are.

I am an interspiritual person myself, born of an unclear mixture of Eastern and Western ancestry as well as Hindu and Christian religious heritage. I found my own identity as both a Hindu and a Christian at an ashram in South India. The late Bede Griffiths, who directed the ashram, Shantivaram, was a rare human being. Clothed in the saffron garb of the Hindu mendicant monk, he remained true to his Christian roots until the end of his life. Yet at the ashram, all the monastic offices began with the chanting of traditional Sanskrit mantras. Father Bede understood the power and beauty of mantra, and he felt that it posed no threat or contradiction to his own Christian roots.

Since mantras represent realities much greater than ourselves, assimilating their power adds to our own greatness, if only we are willing to embrace the magnitude and scope of their possibilities. Yet many are afraid of mantras. Some, recognizing their power, are afraid that they may cause some kind of internal damage, neither noticeable nor curable. Others fear that magical associations implied in these sounds will connect them with witchcraft and sorcery. Then there are those who feel that they would betray their faith in Jesus Christ, or some other personal deity, by using mantras. All of these concerns are legitimate. Every new journey brings understandable fears.

DEITIES AS ENERGY

As we delve into Hindu philosophy, we come to understand that the Hindu Gods and Goddesses are forms of energy. We can see many examples of similar energies around us. Money, for instance, is of course unquestionably worshipped in all places. In spiritual terms, it is a form of energy and can even be seen as a God. What is wonderful about Hinduism is that it gives each form of energy a name and a personality — like our friend Jack, who lives down the street, or our cousin Jane, who are also forms of energy we can approach or refer to by name. Perceived in each form of energy is a governing intelligence — an essence we call "soul." Mantras are sounds that address these essences, awaken us to other presences in the vast field of consciousness, and connect our soul to the energy that emanates from their governing vortexes.

Hindus, like the Celts and Native Americans, perceived personalities in the forms of energy they encountered in nature. Thunder was strong and masculine; water was graceful and feminine; air was mischievous and playful. By attaching symbols to these forms, they better understood their qualities and built relationships with the sources of their energy. Mantras can also be viewed as a form of currency and a means of communication that allow us to exchange energy and intelligence with the unseen world of spiritual presences. Ancient Hindus used mythology, symbols, and sounds to build relationships within the fabric of life. These relationships sustained them emotionally and spiritually.

Yet underlying these symbols for the myriad energies of the universe is, in Hindu philosophy, one great cosmic soul known as Brahman. All other essences and presences are derived from and sustained by this one cosmic entity. As I mentioned in the beginning of this chapter, it was during the first Axial period that the world's religions broke through from the many to the one. In India, the various forms and forces perceived as the many different Gods and Goddesses were now seen as emanations of one Supreme Being: Brahman, derived from the root word *brh,* meaning "to swell." I've always felt that "swelling" of consciousness is a brilliant metaphor for religious experience — the blossoming and expansion of the soul during spiritual awakening.

Brahman, although grammatically neuter in gender, is both beyond and inclusive of gender, and simultaneously conceived of as *Nirguna* and *Saguna.* Nirguna Brahman, which means "reality without attributes," is the transpersonal aspect of the Divine. It transcends attributes altogether, far beyond the normal range of our spiritual perception and the capabilities of mental conception. But when Divinity manifests in the world as creation, it moves through time and takes on form, becoming Saguna, or "with attributes." These accessible attributes of Divine essence are individually venerated through Saguna mantras, which are vibratory representations of Divine energy manifesting in all of creation.

Nirguna and Saguna Mantras

NIRGUNA MANTRAS are mystical statements that connect us directly with the transpersonal and transconceptual Divine absolute. Such a state of consciousness is difficult — even impossible — for many to imagine or conceptualize. But because mantras are exact and specific instruments of spiritual power, it is possible to use them technically, with or without religious belief. One may simply employ their amazing properties through linguistic precision, in the same way that Hatha Yoga can be practiced expertly without any regard for a supreme intelligence. A good example of a Nirguna mantra is the sacred *Gayatri,* listed in appendix one.

Saguna mantras, or mantras embodying attributes, are the form of mantra that often make the non-Hindu uncomfortable because they are addressed to Shiva or Kali or Vishnu or Ram — all multi-armed Hindu Gods and Goddesses with Hindu faces, surrounded by an assortment of exotic symbols. Saguna mantras, such as the mantra *Om Shivaaya Namaha,* refer to individual qualities of the Supreme Being, which are then personalized as Gods or Goddesses with specific functions and qualities. These Saguna mantras allow human beings to access the Divine through understandable attributes. They sometimes awaken resistance, particularly in Christians who may feel that a "false god" is being invoked. More fundamentally, Christians may fear that their God of the Heavens will punish them for flirting with another deity, much as he did in the Old Testament with those who worshipped Baal.

Understanding how Hinduism, in the forms of Nirguna and Saguna, actually parallels the ideas of mystical Christianity can help us overcome these fears. Christian theologian Meister Eckhart explains the difference between Nirguna and Saguna through the terms "God" and "the Godhead." The Godhead, for Eckhart, is like Nirguna Brahman; it is the very essence of reality, at the heart of all existence. We cannot properly speak of it in human language because it is beyond time, beyond space, beyond becoming, beyond death, beyond change, and beyond gender. God, on the other hand, is the Divine intervening in the human situation, perceived through human attributes we can talk about: love, mercy, justice, and compassion. Knowing the many individual aspects of the Divine apart from the One can therefore feel incomplete and be confusing, as is evident in Eckhart's famous prayer, "I ask God to rid me of God." Here, he asks to be free of human projections so that he can "know God, as God is." This is the ultimate move from Saguna Brahman to Nirguna Brahman, and such movement is the natural order of all chants. Paradoxically, with mantras we use words to go beyond words to get to the essence of word itself.

Each vision of Brahman holds its own danger. To stay fixated on the transcendent One, while negating the many aspects and diversity of the Divine, can make for an impersonal spiritual approach that doesn't recognize human frailty and suffering, or in other cases creates a sense of superiority and religious discrimination against others. The other extreme is to become overly engrossed with specific attributes of the Divine in a way that prevents us from penetrating to the depth of Divine essence. The former endangers excessive transcendence, the latter excessive immanence. Our challenge today is to bring together the One and the many in a celebration of the All, a goal that mantra can help us achieve.

Since Hinduism teaches that there is only one Supreme Being with many attributes, it can be conversely stated that any single attribute can lead us back to the One. With this in mind, Hindus regard the sound structure of that attribute (the Saguna mantra) as a sort of hologram — a part that contains the whole, a slice of reality that can lead us back to the One.* Thus, every Saguna mantra is fundamentally an energetic form of some aspect of the Divine. While in Christianity, Islam, and Judaism, the one Almighty God is worshipped by many attributes such as kindness, love, and mercy, Hinduism reverently uses sonic formulae to embody and release these same attributes in our own body and soul. Saguna mantras, therefore, provide us with a means of absorbing Divine attributes into ourselves so that we can increase our own divinity and aspire to our highest good.

ACCEPTING THE POWER OF DEITY MANTRAS

While it is fully permissible to initially choose to maintain mental images when chanting deity mantras, the image in mantra practice must eventually dissolve so that the reality of the mantra's force can come into focus. For instance, some practitioners find it helpful to use an image of Shiva while chanting a Shiva mantra, or an image of Jesus when chanting a Jesus mantra. The ideal method of mantra practice is to allow the patterns of energy that are awakened during mantra recitation to naturally take form in our consciousness. In this manner, the mantra may awaken images from the unconscious or generate kaleidoscopic patterns of energy reflective of the deep transformation in effect during the recitation. Yet our deepest mystical experiences always require that we travel beyond the realm of name and form to that place of deep stillness and silence within us; here, sound and movement manifest as the most subtle vibrations.

Jesus showed his followers that he had to die in order that a new world be born. After his death on the cross, he appeared to his disciples in a spiritual body that defied the laws of this physical world. In the same way, the external mantra, through repeated use, transforms our consciousness into the body of the mantra, a spiritual field that defies the laws of this physical world. All our expectations and images ultimately dissolve in this radical transformation.

I will provide some guidelines here that can help you get accustomed

* There are two schools of Vedic grammarians. For the Sphotavada school, the entire mantra is necessary to awaken inner illumination *(sphota)* because of the interdependence of meaning between words necessary to complete a sentence. The other school, Varnavada, leans toward the Tantric view and stresses that individual letters (*varnas,* which also means caste and form) are capable of awakening the intended illumination.

to using Hindu deity mantras. These methods work equally well for those who are already comfortable with such mantras, as it will help them access deeper experiences through a more meaningful understanding of these sounds.

First, as we've discussed, remind yourself repeatedly to separate the mantra from the visual form of the deity it evokes, which is merely an anthropomorphic representation of a cosmic force. For instance, you may have seen an image of Shiva with a trident in his hand and a snake around his neck; this image may appear in your mind as you chant a Shiva mantra. If this happens, it is important to realize that this is not the actual presence of the vibrational field of intelligence and energy that is represented by the Shiva mantra; rather, it is only one possible variation of the field.

Next, try to discern the archetypal attribute of the Divine that a particular mantra represents. Identifying this broader meaning can help us feel comfortable and confident about using the mantra. Shiva, for instance, means "the beneficent one." So when we use the mantra Shiva, we are addressing an approachable aspect of a terrifying mystery that is ultimately beneficent. Shiva is also the Divine dancer whose motions are the energies of the universe. To use the mantra *Shiva* is to worship the great dance of creation.

Third, endeavor to understand the particular function of the mantra you want to use. For instance, a Shiva mantra can be used to remove fear, particularly the fear of change. In the Hindu Trinity, Shiva is associated with destruction, which is a negative term for the constant restructuring of energy, without which the universe could not organize itself into new forms. With this in mind, we can use Shiva mantras to instill a sense of confidence within us, especially when we are faced with radical changes.

Fourth, learn to interpret the symbols associated with a deity in a meaningful way. We can learn their archetypal value from within their cultural contexts. For instance, in the Hindu yogic tradition, the snake around Shiva's neck represents spiritual consciousness; the goal of the yogi is to awaken spiritual consciousness, hence the image of the serpent with a raised head. Understanding the symbols associated with a particular mantra can therefore become an energetic stimulant in our practice.

Once you have accepted the energetic power of the symbol, you can mentally use it as a spiritual container for the mantra. This is particularly helpful if you are a visually oriented person. If you are more kinesthetic — oriented toward your physical body and its movement — you might use the symbol in the form of an amulet or pendant to wear on your body. External symbols and objects associated with mantra practice act as sponges that soak up the vibrations of the recitation. Such empowered objects can then be offered to others so that they can be affected by the vibrations of the mantra. This is the Tantric way.

Hindus like to use images that they can bathe, touch, and anoint while reciting mantras. Many Hindus worship the noniconic form of Shiva — the lingam — which symbolizes a pillar of light and can represent a formless aspect of the Divine. (The common phallic association of the lingam is often offensive to Hindus, who do not all perceive it that way.) To again find interspiritual comparisons, we can see the close parallel between Shiva and Yahweh, the God of the Old Testament. You may recall the pillar of light that followed the Israelites through the desert, a sign of the Divine protection that accompanied them.

Having said all this, and recognizing the importance of religious context, we must also remember that neither a tactile nor a visual representation is required to awaken the power and technology of mantras. The sound form in itself carries all the resources necessary to generate the desired result, as we will explore in coming chapters. It is our own body, mind, and consciousness that should be affected and transformed by the power of the mantra. However, using mantras can stir up these powerful images and symbols from the unconscious, so it is helpful to understand them rather than fear them. These cultural images can motivate us to discover the power of mantras at an archetypal level of our being, for it is there that the healing power of the mantra is at its peak.

CHAPTER 5

THE SANSKRIT MANTRA

We know that mantras are traditionally spoken or chanted in the Sanskrit language. But can mantras exist in other languages? Can English words, or the sounds of other languages, function as mantras? While it is possible to use any language in a mantric manner by repeating certain patterns, cadences, and inflections, Sanskrit mantras hold a special power. We've touched on some of that power in previous chapters, but here we'll examine Sanskrit and look at what actually happens when we use mantras.

The word for classical Sanskrit comes from the term *Samskrita,* meaning, "well put together." It describes a refined, sculpted technology of sound that was systematically applied to language and phonetics. Linguists have deduced that a root language, which they call Proto-Indo-European, serves as the basis of most great languages and language groups of the Western world. Sanskrit is notably the closest to such a root language. The use of Sanskrit can therefore awaken us to our common spiritual heritage and connect us to each other through an intimate resonance of sacred sound.

"The Sanskrit language, whatever be its antiquity, is of a wonderful structure; more perfect than the Greek, more copious than the Latin, and more exquisitely refined than either, yet bearing to both of them a stronger affinity, both in the roots of verbs and in the forms of grammar, than could possibly have been produced by accident; so strong, indeed, that no philosopher could examine them all three, without believing them to have sprung from some common source, which, perhaps, no longer exists."[1] These words were spoken by Sir William Jones (1746–1794) on February 2, 1786, at an address to the Asiatic Society of Calcutta. Jones was a great scholar and visionary who invented the system of transliteration. He translated the ancient Hindu code of laws known as the laws of Manu (Manusmriti) from Sanskrit into English. He was also the first Westerner to study and write a paper on Indian classical music.[2]

The lost roots of Sanskrit are apparently still in existence but protected by yogic adepts who live deep in the Himalayas. In his book *Living with the Himalayan Masters,*[3] the late Swami Rama describes Sanskrit as having been derived from *Sandhya Basha,* the language of yogic union used to transmit and preserve spiritual experiences within secret yogic schools. This ancient language of prayer, developed by the Himalayan Rishis, is evidently still used among some extraordinary teachers hidden in those mysterious mountains. Sanskrit, too, evolved to communicate and awaken spiritual experience.

FIELDS OF ENERGY

SANSKRIT MANTRAS are like simple energy; they can neither be created nor destroyed; they simply "exist" in the universe. Conversely, the mantras utilized by the yogi serve to awaken the states of meditative awareness encountered by the Rishis so that the actual vibratory field represented by those particular mantras can be experienced.

Although mantras have been codified using Sanskrit, the mantras are themselves beyond the scope of language. They are luminous presences of auditory energy that simply exist in the universe, like vast and pervasive galaxies. The Rishis both saw and heard these fields while in states of deep meditation after having used rigorous yoga practices to enhance their vision and perception, like astronomers polishing the lenses of their telescopes.

When we use Sanskrit mantras, our normal perception of the world dissolves and we awaken to the spiritual fields of energy represented by the sounds. Sanskrit, as a spiritual language, has been accurately and uninterruptedly transmitted for at least four thousand years. The resonance of these sounds uttered by millions of people who have been awakened to spiritual reality assists us in our own use of the language. In other words, we draw from the power of numbers when we use Sanskrit; we connect our soul to numerous yogis and spiritual teachers who have employed this language in their own self-transformation.

GOING BEYOND EVERYDAY CONSCIOUSNESS

The word "mantra" comes from the root *manas,* which refers to the linear, thinking mind. *Tram* means "to protect," "to free," and "to go across." Thus, mantras are sonic formulae that take us beyond, or through, the discursive faculties of the mind and connect our awareness directly and immediately to deep states of energy and consciousness. This capacity of mantra to be both pre-rational and trans-rational can be unsettling for some of us, as we are taught not to trust anything beyond the scope of our five senses. The disquieting, mysterious ancientness of Sanskrit mantras is attributable to the fact that they are not derived from everyday consciousness; they are, in fact, the fruit of spiritual practice (yoga) and spiritual vision. They exemplify the dictum of Jesus to be "in the world, but not of it."

Mantras remind us of spiritual realities that we've banished from our secular world. This is why a language such as English, or any other form of the vernacular, does not help us penetrate beyond the thinking, describing mind to discover spiritual realities. Such languages limit us to the types of consciousness and references that arise from the five sensory organs, or the personality. Our spiritual being, or soul, as Gary Zukav eloquently pointed out in his book *Seat of the Soul,*[4] is multisensory and multidimensional. That is why we need a language such as Sanskrit to capture the complexity of our deeper nature. It doesn't make sense to use the language of the analyzing mind to cut through its own illusions, so we employ the discipline of sonic yoga to balance the limitations of our thinking, describing, analyzing mind.

The *Arthasastra,* a Hindu text from perhaps the third or fourth century A.D., holds that "a mantra accomplishes the apprehension of what is not or cannot be seen, imparts the strength of a definite conclusion to what is apprehended, removes doubt when two courses are possible, and leads to inference of an entire matter when only a part of it is seen."[5]

Sanskrit mantras demonstrate the fact that we can suspend the process of thinking without destroying the rational mind. While critical reason remains alert, we participate in the process of knowing without providing a running commentary. This is the secret of mantra: we are undistracted. But in order to extract the states of consciousness accessible through a mantra, we must first be willing to sacrifice our projections and our descriptions of reality.

CHEMICALS OF THE SOUL

Sanskrit is largely a language of prayer, yoga, and ritual. Indeed, it includes many words for spiritual experiences and concepts that have no equivalents in other languages. Recognizing this linguistic precision, we must then recognize that a key component of a Sanskrit mantra is therefore its pronunciation. When attention is paid to this detail, the power of the mantra is magnified. Unfortunately, many Western yogis ignore this crucial component of mantra by claiming that your intention is all that counts. That is the equivalent of your Hatha Yoga teacher telling you that sloppy posture is alright. Pronunciation forms the backbone of mantra, which strengthens the infrastructure of the soul. The pronunciation of Sanskrit actually carries with it an astonishingly sensual experience — a lively exploration of the mouth with the tongue that stimulates energy both spiritually and sexually.

The hard and soft palate, as noted earlier, are a blueprint of the body's nervous system. Sound yogis use this knowledge to manipulate the body's spiritual channels in much the same way that a reflexologist uses the hands and feet to stimulate the body's meridians. Dr. Dharma Singh Khalsa, whom I quoted in chapter one, mentions the existence of sixty-four meridian points on the hard palate, and twenty meridian points on the soft palate.[6] Stimulating these points, especially through the rich phonetics of Sanskrit, effects powerful changes in the pituitary gland and the hypothalamus, which govern our immune system, our emotions, and our moods. This is why medical research continues to confirm the assertion that chanting produces beneficial chemicals in the body, releasing "feel-good" hormones and endorphins, the body's natural painkillers.

Dr. Khalsa points out that chanting yogic mantras, particularly in Sanskrit, stimulates the vagus nerve, which is situated near the jaw and is considered to be the single most important nerve in the body; it services the heart, lungs, intestinal tract, and back muscles. Sanskrit, because of its complex consonants, stimulates an enormous quantity of energy in the body and in the spiritual nervous system.

So what does proper pronunciation of Sanskrit phonetics involve? Most important is the correct positioning of the tongue in the mouth and the proper articulation of compound consonants. The difference between a poorly pronounced mantra and a correctly pronounced one is comparable to the difference between a movie and real life: the former can only simulate an effect; the latter is the real thing.

The subtlety of activating specific meridian points through proper pronunciation is further illustrated in the words of noted mantra scholar Harvey Alper. As Alper explains, "Each mantra is understood to be a finely honed instrument for exercising power, a tool designed for a particular task, which will achieve a specific spiritual purpose when and only when used in a particular manner."[7] Without correct pronunciation, the practitioner is denied access to the intended power of the mantra. This is especially true of Tantric bijas (*lam, vam,* and so on) and Vedic mantras, such as the sacred *Gayatri* mantra *(Om, Bhur, Bhuvas, Suvaha),* which are performed with tremendous liberties in yoga and chanting performances today. On the downloadable audio tracks that accompany this book, I will provide a pronunciation guide that corresponds with the appendixes. As I will explain in chapter nine, devotional mantras are an exception to rules of pronunciation, although their power can be enhanced through the basic applications of pronunciation guidelines.

SEEING WITH THE THIRD EYE

The use of Sanskrit mantras helps awaken the third eye, or *ajna* chakra, which is the command center positioned between the eyebrows. As Jesus said, "Let your eye be single." This unified vision is awakened only when the discursive, linear brain is suspended.

As I mentioned earlier, the Rishis of ancient India both "saw" and "heard" mantras in their meditations. This crossing-over of faculties is not difficult to understand. Dr. Larry Dossey uses the term *synesthetes* to describe individuals in whom multiple senses operate simultaneously

— for example, people who can smell sounds or see musical tones. The gift of seeing sound even has a Sanskrit name: *Mantra Dhrista.*

Such experiences are beyond the ordinary modes of perception common to our everyday consciousness. They are available to us when we rise above our normal, habituated modes of perception — above the viewpoints others want us to employ. We may unconsciously choose such habitual modes because they feel comfortable, or because those we love and respect see things that way, or because we are tricked into seeing and believing this way because it is advantageous to someone else, notably through certain forms of popular media and advertising.

The use of Sanskrit mantras may be invaluable in our times, helping us develop our own special perspective in a culture that constantly bombards us with information. Sanskrit mantras help us rise beyond the habits of normal perception to a realm where, like a phoenix, we awaken to something fuller, richer, more expansive, more beautiful, and more magnificent than what is typically present in our everyday consciousness. Obviously, this is something we all need a dose of every day — a perceptual tonic. Otherwise, we easily become overwhelmed with the details of everyday life, and we forget the vastness of inner spaces available to the soul.

Many of us secretly suffer from psychic claustrophobia and don't know what to do about it. Sanskrit mantras can help us break through our psychological prisons. Conveniently, mantras can be utilized anywhere: in the middle of a traffic jam, in an elevator, or even in the midst of a business meeting. All we need to do is train ourselves to use these mantras effectively.

CHAPTER 6

BUILDING OUR SONIC COMMUNITY

How many mantras do we really need? Where do we start? Do we need a guru or realized soul to impart our mantra to us? How do we build a mantra vocabulary? This chapter addresses these questions.

I am often asked in my workshops and seminars if we need to receive our mantras from a guru. Traditionally, a mantra is imparted to a yogi or mantra practitioner by an enlightened soul — someone who has realized the power of a particular mantra. Often, this special sound was handed down to the teacher by his or her own guru, creating an unbroken chain of energy. Such a mantra is like a vessel that never runs dry, but is handed over from one person to another.

But today a more common, practical method is a self-initiatory process of working with a specific selection of mantras. I believe that this is by far the most powerful method, and one that is most needed now. In this approach, individuals prepare their mind, heart, and body with their own set of self-empowering mantras. These mantras then become their "sonic community." This is the method I will be sharing with you.

In ancient times, mantras were tightly controlled and administered under specific conditions. This was necessary to protect both the mantras and the practitioners from misusing these sacred instruments of power. Today, our need for mantras is urgent. Bringing the energy of the spiritual realm into our physical reality is crucial in order to compensate for the great banishment of the sacred from our culture. Mantras are catalysts of spiritual transformation, and they must be made available to as many people as possible.

Those who wish to receive their mantras from an enlightened soul should definitely do so. In the Hindu tradition, there are three types of guides: God, guru, and *acharya.* "God" usually refers to any spiritual force or being of light — an angel, a deity, or an ancient power. An acharya is a teacher or spiritual guide, while a guru is an enlightened soul, either living or passed on from the body. Although gurus that meet all our expectations may be hard to find in this day and age, they still exist. And a spiritual guide can always point the way. At the same time, I believe that we have to stop projecting our own enlightenment onto other people. We must learn to trust in our own light, believe in our own spiritual potencies, and stop worrying excessively about getting things right the first time.

The Buddha said:

Believe nothing because a wise person said it,
Believe nothing because it is generally held.
Believe nothing because it is written.
Believe nothing because it is said to be Divine.
Believe nothing because someone else believes it.
But believe only what you yourself judge to be true.[1]

OUR CORE MANTRA

IN DEVELOPING a community of mantras, the most important mantra of all is our core mantra. This is the mantra that many receive from their guru. Our core mantra addresses the essential dimension of being: our innermost Self, our deepest spiritual nature, our soul.

Our core mantra affirms the alignment of our soul with the Divine ground of existence; it should instantly awaken us to the highest, greatest, most powerful, most authentic, most wise, most beautiful, and most inspiring awareness of Spirit in our memory. The key word is "resonance" or, more precisely, "multidimensional resonance." The realm of the five senses is the realm of the personality, constructed and oriented by an education in this world and limited to knowledge of this world. Multidimensional resonance is the awakening of all our senses, including the spiritual senses: intuition, spiritual vision and knowledge, awareness of life's blessings, trust in Divine providence, and the fullness of love, peace, and joy.

It is preferable to avoid choosing our core mantra in the language we think in. Complex prayers like the rosary and the Lord's Prayer may function well as mantric prayers, provided they do not get the thinking mind into gear. I personally find the rosary and the Lord's Prayer deeply meaningful; they allow me to sense the Divine presence in a profound way, particularly when I think about what the words mean. For precisely that reason, I don't use them in mantra recitation.

Also, our core mantra is not used to speak to God, stimulate intellectual ideas, or provoke reflection on spiritual matters. Reflective prayer is necessary, and so are conversations with God, but they must be reserved for other times. "Mantra is meaningful, not in any descriptive or even persuasive sense," explains mantra scholar Bharati Ageananda. "It is verifiable not by what it describes, but what it effects."[2]

To hone our core mantra's power to affect our consciousness, the mantra should be short: a single word or phrase to summon the Divine presence. It may be as simple as the mantra Om. If you want to use a Christian mantra form, you might try adding the name of Jesus to the mantra: *Ye-su Om,* or *Om Namah Christaaya,* which is the Sanskrit form of "I worship the presence of Christ as the Divine Word through which all things are created."

The repeated sounding of our core mantra reinforces the capacity of soul to express itself fully in our personality — to incarnate. The personality, which repeatedly hears this mantra, opens like a flower and accommodates the authentic expressions of our soul, working with it rather than against it. Our core mantra moves us toward wholeness because the repeated sounding of the mantra pulls together the disparate portions of our being.

Our core mantra also helps remove fear, proving to be our true salvation at the moment of death. When a mantra achieves this level of depth, it becomes our *aabhath* mantra — a sound capable of rescuing us from all perils and dangers. This mantra will spontaneously come to our attention at the moment of death, helping us find our way home to our source in the Divine. Gandhi, when he was shot, died uttering his core mantra *Ram,* a popular name for the Divine in India. *Ram* mystically signifies "that which awakens joy in the heart." Our core mantra should therefore be synonymous with our deepest experience of the Divine since it is to be used most of the time, during meditation, and particularly in times of stress or danger.

OUR RECOVERY MANTRA

As many of us quickly discover in spiritual practice, the path is about love. But until we have discovered the connection between our soul and the Great Spirit of the Universe, and sensed the role of our personality in the midst of it all, the spiritual path is more about technique than relationship. The essence of the spiritual life — or, for that matter, life itself — is love. But because love cannot reach its full stature and depth without complete freedom, it isn't easy for us to remain uninterruptedly aligned with the core of our being. We repeatedly lose this connection through our obstinacy, egocentricity, impatience, and anger.

In the past, many spiritual teachers have said, "Just say your mantra, whatever is going on inside you." Yet I have noticed that whenever we fall from our natural state of grace, saying our core mantra feels insincere. We know that we aren't aligned with the core of our being, and it's no use pretending that we are. For this reason, I recommend having a recovery mantra. Our recovery mantra functions as a purifying device because it acknowledges that we've fallen into egocentricity and affirms that we need grace to help us out of it. This complementary sacred formula proves indispensable in helping us maintain balance.

In the more advanced stages of our mantra *sadhana* (spiritual discipline), it may be possible to reduce all our meditations to a single sound, a single breath, or a single movement. To get to that point, however, we may need many sounds, many breaths, and many movements. Our progression, therefore, is from the many to the One.

It may appear that our recovery mantra is a bit circuitous, but it is very effective. Here's an example: Some of my most challenging situations manifest when I make decisions with my wife. As with most couples, I find it especially difficult with her to give up my opinions, admit that I'm wrong, or simply not get my way. When this happens, I feel like some of the best parts of myself have been squeezed out of their deep center. Then, depending on how inflated my ego gets, I have a hard time readjusting to my core. You may nod knowingly or relate to the same conditions with your coworker, your boss, or some of your clients. Each of us has vulnerable circuits that feed back into our consciousness, and the situations that trigger them may run into the hundreds — even thousands — each month.

During such times, my core mantra lacks efficacy. Even though I'm saying my core mantra, there is a mad rush of activity going on in my mind and emotions. It's possible to wait out this flurry of thought and emotion, but often that seems to take forever. During such phases, I have found that my recovery mantra, *Naaraayana, Naaraayana* ("Oh perfect One, come to my assistance"), uttered with great fervor, helps me regain the connection I've lost. This mantra reminds me, through its simple formula, that I am dwelling too strongly in my ego and that I'm being too self-reliant or judgmental. It also has a soothing sound, which helps me work my way back to the core of my being more quickly and effectively than hammering my emotions with my core mantra. You, of course, should find the mantra that produces this effect for you.

In Christian terms, the recovery mantra is similar to asking for forgiveness or assistance; it helps keep us honest and humble. There are still occasions when I use "Lord, have mercy on me" as a recovery mantra. For a non-Christian, or for someone who doesn't want to relate to a personalized form of the Divine, a recovery mantra needn't literally state "God, please forgive me," but it can be a sound or phrase that conveys a sense of humility in its energetic resonance. This mantric resonance expresses — without explicit words — a desire to reconnect with our highest truth. For instance, the mantra *Sharanam Ananda, Satchidananda* can be used as a recovery mantra. It means "I seek refuge in the Being, knowledge, and bliss of spiritual reality." You can find other appropriate mantras in the appendixes.

I find that a set of mantric syllables is far more effective than a phrase in English or whatever one's "thinking language" may be; it bypasses the mind's tendency to reflect on the phrase and directly addresses the emotional dynamics of our energy. The rhythm of the mantra cohesively draws together the disparate streams of energy caused by our negligence and helps us recover our connection to the essence of our being. I sometimes use *Om Maha Deviye Namaha,* a Sanskrit phrase that can be translated as, "Great Mother, make haste to help me."

From another practical standpoint, the repeated use of our core mantra — or any other single sound — can easily dull our awareness and cause us to tune out; our recovery mantra serves to maintain contrast and balance in our Yoga of Sound practice. Almost all television stations worldwide alternate between male and female voices in their news broadcasts; this helps maintain viewers' attention through gender balance and vocal contrast. Likewise, our own alternation between a core mantra and a recovery mantra helps us maintain a strong connection to the core of our being. We recognize that the ego is always present, and we keep it transparent through the use of the recovery mantra. Using the core mantra and recovery mantra in a healthy balance, and within proper contexts, helps strengthen our mental and emotional reflexes.

BUILDING OUR MANTRA COMMUNITY

Rooted in our core mantra and balanced with our recovery mantra, we are strong enough to create around ourselves an entire community of mantras that fortify our soul. This extended vocabulary of sacred sounds will continually support and strengthen us, much like taking our daily vitamin supplements does. Also, just as there is tremendous strength in having constant support from a group of human beings who truly understand and support our spiritual path, our community of mantras fortifies our soul when human beings are unavailable. Whenever we feel alone on the path, our community of mantras creates a net of safety around us and assists us in whatever spiritual process we are undergoing at that time.

Another perspective is that our community of mantras represents those Divine attributes and qualities that we seek to develop in ourselves. Catholics have a wonderful tradition of praying to the saints. Developing a community of mantras is similar to believing in a "communion of saints." When approaching the saints, Catholics generally perceive these presences as dwelling outside the range of their consciousness, in heaven. Through intercessory prayer, Catholics reach out to these saints and draw them into their field of awareness, asking for their intervention. Being closer to God than we are, the saint is considered more capable of directing Divine power toward an event or situation. In the same way, through mantras we can come into immediate contact with the power we need in our lives; the sound actually contains the necessary force and links us directly to a reservoir full of that power. As we sound the mantra in our body, we channel this power into the desired situation or area in our lives. The power, in this case, is inside us.

How, then, do we start to build our community of mantras? We are so accustomed to having our lives well-packaged that we might expect to find mantra manuals listing ingredients and instructions. But as mantra practitioners, we must season our spiritual channels much as we might season a cooking pan; only then can we truly taste the energy of mantras and realize their intended effect upon us. Otherwise, this food for our soul can stick to the pan or just not cook to perfection.

A regular practice of mantra, incorporating the elements of Sound Yoga as described in part four, is essential to this seasoning process; it helps us understand and work with mantras efficiently. As you read this book and work with the accompanying audio tracks, you will begin to understand mantras and their applications on a deeper level. Over time, you will build your community of mantras. I have provided a reference at the end of this chapter to give you a sense of how this might come together, but you must develop your own relationship with mantras to build your own unique force field.

The same mantra, for instance, may have different effects on different people, or it may vary its effects on the same person in different times or situations. This does not mean that there aren't specific mantras for specific purposes. On the contrary, there are vast quantities of mantras for specific purposes, from the curing of snakebite to forcing someone to fall in love with you. Of course, if such mantras worked for everyone, I would be a wealthy man and so would millions of other Indians. What makes the mantra effective is belief, or faith. We believe something because it rings true in our depths; faith gives us the energy to act on that belief.

During a break at one of my conferences, a bald man came up to me and seriously asked, "Do you have a mantra that can grow hair?" A mischievous Sufi friend of mine who was standing nearby replied just as seriously, "If you chant 'Hairy Krishna' with the belief that your hair will grow, I guarantee that it will." Humorous though this situation was, it is true that belief and faith can manifest anything we want — even move mountains if need be. The real mountains, though, are the blocks in our spiritual lives and our energy systems that can be dissolved through the proper use of mantras.

The inner life is a type of spiritual archeology. This is why, to aid us in our faith and belief, mantras have been sculpted and refined into sophisticated tools for the soul. Also, what makes a mantra work is not just the sound itself, but all the preparation involved: our mental and physical framework, our environment, our interpretation, our self-talk, any ritualistic aspects we use, our attunement to the sounds, the inflections we use, and so on. Chapter eleven covers many of these key principles of preparation and presents many applications of mantra shastra that can assist you in your efforts.

PUTTING IT ALL TOGETHER

When we explore our inner world and discover the vast landscape of consciousness, it can be empowering to carry a community of spiritual forces with us as we move from region to region. As our spiritual life takes us across diverse terrains, our core mantra functions as a staff that offers constant and immediate support. When we are distracted, our recovery mantra acts as a compass, helping us return to the path. When we are lonely or in need of extra protection, our community of mantras is there to assist us. All too often, the spiritual life has been described as a lonely path; with mantras, it needn't be so.

In this age of spiritual curiosity, an assortment of mantras may sound alluring. Your own experimentation will reveal that limiting your spiritual practice to a collection of mantras without regularly practicing a core mantra will not effectively bank the spiritual energy generated by your practice; it only assuages a superficial need for spiritual consciousness. Indiscriminately using a set of mantras without a proper context neither builds confidence nor takes the user to a truly deep place. Following the principles and techniques described in subsequent chapters will help you derive unlimited power from the Yoga of Sound tradition.

We want to build a community of mantras, not a collection of mantras. To achieve this, keep in mind that all mantras should be used for a substantial period of time so that their effects can be absorbed. Consistent effort should be invested in the proper pronunciation of the mantra, which should be refined over time. Above all, proper preparation, a conducive environment, conscientious diet, and focused intention will reliably take you to the heights of the Yoga of Sound. Once again, you will find all this information in chapter eleven.

A COMMUNITY OF MANTRAS

THE FOLLOWING SET of mantras will give you an idea of what it means to have a community of mantras. The meaning of these mantras and their pronunciation can be found in the appendixes, which will also explain their specific functions. You will, of course, evolve your own set of mantras that resonate with your personality. Your mantras may change with the phases of your life — roughly once in every seven years — but this change is not something you should deliberately seek.

Core mantra: *Om Na-mah Shi-vaa-ya*
Recovery mantra: *Om Shaan-ti, Shaan-ti, Shaan-ti Om*
To remove fear: *Om Kshroum Na-ra-shim-haa-ya Na-ma-ha*
To invite abundance: *Om Shring Ma-haa Laksh-mi-ye Na-ma-ha*
To clear obstacles: *Om Gam Ga-na-pa-tai-ye Namaha*
To enhance our relationships: *Om Kleem Krish-Naa-ya Namaha*
For inspiration and creativity: *Om Aim Sa-ras-wa-tai-ye Namaha*
For our professional lives: *Om Namo Naa-raa-ya-naa-ya*
For morning praise: the *Gayatri* mantra
For noon practice: Bija mantras for the chakras

For evening praise: *Shri Raa-ma, Jai Raa-ma, Jai, Jai, Raa-mo*
At night: *So Ham*

Most of these mantras are used only for short periods during the day; choose the timing and duration based on your needs to achieve specific goals or resolve particular situations. Throughout the day and night, we use our core mantra to stay connected to our essence, and whenever necessary we use our recovery mantra to reestablish that connection when dulled or broken. During times of illness or when disruptions occur, we may resort to therapeutic mantras that help remedy a particular situation. Like therapeutic diets, we don't use these special mantras on a regular basis.

Awake! Arise! Strive for the highest and be in the light. Sages say that the path is narrow and difficult to tread — as narrow as the edge of a razor.

Katha Upanishad[3]

PART 3

TRADITION

THE FOUR MAJOR STREAMS OF SACRED SOUND IN HINDUISM

Shabda Yoga for strength

Shakti Yoga for energy

Bhava Yoga for relationship

Nada Yoga for harmony

CHAPTER 7

SHABDA YOGA:
THE SPIRITUAL TECHNOLOGY OF VEDIC MANTRAS

The idea of the power of the word is as old as the Vedas of the Hindus.

— ***Hazrat Inayat Khan,* The Mysticism of Sound and Music**[1]

The first stream of Sound Yoga we will explore is Shabda Yoga, which can be translated as "word yoga." Although "shabda" refers to the spoken, "sounded," or uttered word, it may be worth applying the principles of shabda to the written word as well, since a word is sounded in our minds as we read or write. We may further extend our use of *word* to include electronic communications such as e-mail, bringing the ancient principles of this stream of Sound Yoga into some of the most important activities of our present lives.

THE POWER OF SOUND MADE VISIBLE

The effect of words on our consciousness and on the material world has been made visible through the amazing work of Japanese scientist Masuro Emoto. In 1992, Dr. Emoto, a quantum physicist from

Yokohama, performed a series of experiments on water crystals around the world. These experiments revealed the astonishing fact that water is receptive to external messages communicated through sound. These communications may be spoken through human language, written by means of printed characters, played as music, or even thought in the mind — a testimony to the power of the word as shabda, and also to sound as nada.

Positive messages — kind thoughts or positive words such as "love" and "thank you" — actually purified the water. The effect was visible as beautiful hexagonal patterns formed in the water crystals. The same thing happened when the water was exposed to classical music, such as Bach's Goldberg variations. In contrast, water exposed to cruel thoughts, heavy-metal music, or negative printed characters (for example, words such as "Hitler" or even "you fool" written and pasted on a bottle of water) formed water crystals of a distorted and chaotic shape.[2]

Emoto's work provides us with evidence that human energy in the form of thoughts, words, ideas, and music has a vibrational quality that affects the molecular structure of water. When we reflect on the fact that our physical bodies consist of about 70 percent water, and that an equal percentage of the earth's surface is water, we begin to get a sense of the magnitude of this discovery. We have tremendous power to affect our health and well-being in positive, powerful ways through our words.

In the language of psychology, water is a symbol of the unconscious mind. In the Bible, water was associated with the Divine body; the first line of Genesis begins with "In the beginning, the Spirit of God hovered over the waters." For thousands of years, water has been the primary ritual ingredient for Hindu people; many forms of mantra using water are employed today. Imagine, then, the power of mantras as words of transformation and their ability to affect our physical and mental consciousness. From Emoto's research, we realize that our words and sounds not only affect our own bodies, but also the bodies of other living organisms, which also contain water. It is therefore possible for us to consciously transform the world if we believe and trust in the power of our words.

Another key figure is Dr. Larry Dossey, who was instrumental in waking up the medical world to the sound of prayer and its ability to affect health, life, and consciousness. Dr. Dossey found that prayer was effective regardless of whether the subject believed in the process or not and regardless of the distance involved. The fact that our words have the power to affect life so deeply should inspire us to refine our sound, our voice, and our personal vibration field. This is the value of practicing Shabda Yoga.

THE MYSTERY OF THE DIVINE WORD

To understand the power of the spoken word, it is necessary to compare our own capacity to utter words with the creative power of the Divine to manifest the universe. The opening verse of St. John's gospel sums up this Divine power:

In the beginning was the Word;
the word was with God,
and the word was God.

The first phrase states the obvious: that the origin of the universe was a great word, a great thought in the Divine mind. Secondly, this massive quantity of energy was "with God." One interpretation is that this word was inside God, just waiting to exhale. It can also mean that the Word was pregnant with purpose and potential. Finally, there is the powerful conclusion that the word "was God." Here we understand the Word as the supreme expression of the Divine, as the thought of God, synonymous with the Divine Presence and therefore *being* God. We see an amazing consortium of vibratory power present in the Word — a great potentiality and creative power that is synonymous with Divine presence. For the Christian, this is the mystery of the Holy Trinity. It also sums up the goal of the sound yogi, for whom the Word is used to merge with the Sonic Absolute — Shabda Brahman — in such a manner that the mind of the yogi, the process of yoga, and the object of yoga — samadhi consciousness — become unified as one indivisible whole.

The mysticism of the word is especially apt. On the human level, we know that breath is required in order to produce words. Thus, all of creation is produced and sustained by the breath of God. St. Thomas Aquinas drew from this vision when he wrote: "All creatures are words of God, and all of creation is a book about God." In the chapter of Genesis, the ancient Hebrew word *ruah* was used to describe the "breath" of God that hovered over the primal waters of creation. It was with this breath that the first creative Divine intentions were spoken. Each spoken intention manifested as reality: "God *said,* 'Let there be light,' and there was light."

Our intentions, too, can manifest into reality, provided that they come from that deep place where we are absolutely one with the Divine — with Truth — and provided that what we desire is for the good of the universe. The light shines upon all without discrimination; the earth allows all to walk upon her without distinction; and water cleanses all without prejudice. So to be like the Divine is to want good for the world, and to want it without distinction. Yet even when we fall short of this level of altruism, the power of speech to manifest reality is so great that even evil intent, which can be described as misdirected good, is also capable of manifesting into reality.

From the story of Genesis, we are also told that the Divine transfers its vitality and essence into the clay by "breathing into it." Such mythological images further attest to the tremendous creative power that can be associated with breath and with sacred utterance. Add the fact that many native cultures have the same linguistic roots for "dance" as they do for "breath," and we begin to see the world as dancing words, as poetry and music.

MANIFESTING OUR OWN UNIVERSE

Shabda Yoga teaches us that we can learn to manifest our own universe if we apply the principles outlined in St. John's gospel. These principles were well understood and practiced by the ancient Vedic seers and Rishis, who were also great poets. Vedic mantras, which are the classic form of Shabda Yoga, are well-sculpted poetic nuances. Another form of Shabda Yoga is poetry from around the world. Rap music, too, can be a type of Shabda Yoga if it is employed with yogic consciousness and the intention of transforming the world, rather than as an unbridled outlet for negative energy and frustration.

Present-day motivational speakers and self-help authors have drawn attention to this age-old understanding of the power of human speech to manifest our dreams, our desires, and our fears. They teach us to change self-negating thoughts into positive affirmations in order to create more wealth and success in our lives. Much of what we think does, in fact, manifest into reality.

Imagine, then, that we widen the scope of this possibility beyond personal wealth and ambition to include profound matters of the soul. Imagine that we can draw energy from the sound of animals and birds, the stars, the sun, and the moon. Imagine channeling all that energy into our own nervous system. We would be able to build an immense reservoir of power to transform our families, our communities, our planet, and ourselves with the same power we have been seeking outside ourselves. Shabda Yoga is an age-old system that is a spiritual technology of the soul, a system already in use that can be expanded to create a better world for us all.

KEY PRINCIPLES OF SHABDA YOGA

The principles of Shabda Yoga are based on the spiritual power of words. These principles are:

- The sound of the word truly represents the sound of the thing it is associated with.
- There is an irrefutable sense of truth in the word and the sound.
- The composite structure of the words in a sentence or a group of sentences awakens spiritual illumination.
- A force-field of energy is generated by employing the rhythmic meters of intoning the words.
- The sounds establish energetic connections among the user, the listener, and thing signified.

Traditional Vedic mantras are a sophisticated form of spiritual poetry that captures the emotional intensity and articulate beauty of the Sanskrit language. Many Vedic mantras have gone through a rigorous process of refinement in order to embody the principles listed. This process includes not only the meaning of the words but also their phonetic beauty, which embodies an innate music that can awaken the soul to knowledge, spiritual vision, and insight. Such an awakening is possible when words work together in a sentence structure to simultaneously capture the intellect, the imagination, and the full scope of human emotion. Thus, Vedic mantras reveal a cosmic vision by awakening spiritual insight in the user as well as in the listener.

The Vedas, which are composed mostly of Vedic mantras, are considered to have been birthed from two inseparable aspects: *sruti* (that which is heard) and *smriti* (that which is remembered). One way of understanding these aspects of Vedic mantras is that the words and sounds awaken memory — knowledge that is already encoded in our cells, genes, and DNA. The combination of meaning and rhythm in Vedic mantras, arranged in specific sentence structures and poetic meters, serves to illuminate the soul, especially when chanted during ritual. It was within the context of ancient Vedic rituals that these mantras were developed.

Vedic mantras are often recited aloud. The word "mantra" is derived from the ancient Vedic word *manas,* representing the mind, and *tra* meaning "instrumentality." A mantra is therefore an instrument of the mind, a spiritual device capable of producing transformation. A lesser-known interpretation of the word "mantra" comes from the root *man-a,* meaning "to utter." This explains Vedic mantras and Shabda Yoga as a form of sacred speech that must be spoken aloud, as in the recitation of sacred texts, so that it could be "heard by the Gods." Since speech causes our thoughts to manifest into reality, Vedic mantras — used to negotiate with the Gods — were painstakingly sculpted and refined so that even the Gods could not refuse what was being asked of them.

The function of linking human aspirations with the Divine power of the universe to fulfill these aspirations leads us to yet another aspect of Vedic mantras: clarity of speech. The Vedic priest is very articulate in his enunciation of mantras so that the utterance is decisive — even aggressive. Thus, Shabda Yoga constitutes what we might classify as a masculine approach to Sound Yoga. For many thousands of years, women were not taught these mantras. In our present situation, I believe it is imperative that women be introduced to this type of chanting so that they can reclaim their voice and power. Such a step moves us toward the balance we are seeking as a culture and as a species.

The masculine power and articulate structure of Vedic mantras are best utilized to instill strength and confidence. It is therefore practical to use such sounds in the morning as we prepare for the day's tasks.

They can also be used during the day when we feel our confidence being depleted or whenever we feel vulnerable, because shabda mantras fortify our spiritual presence and give us power. Even if you weren't using Sanskrit mantras, you can feel the power of words by articulating what you want. Using Sanskrit mantras will bolster your regular speech and thinking abilities many times over.

The Vedic grammarians emphasized two aspects of the word (shabda), namely *dhvani* and *sphota*. Dhvani is the articulated external sound we hear with our ears; sphota is the inner, illuminating power awakened in the heart when the word is "heard right." In order for this to happen, speech must be articulate and syntax properly constructed. When we go deeply into this process, we allow the power of language to transmit insight and remove ignorance. Language then becomes a guru, capable of dispelling the darkness and illuminating the soul with its light. According to the philosophical Hindu text *Advayatarака Upanishad,* "guru" means "dispeller" *(gu)* of "darkness" *(ru)*.[3]

THE GODDESS OF SACRED SPEECH

In ancient languages, the sound of a word contained the energy and essence of the thing signified by that word. The earliest forms of communication were probably grunts, groans, screams, and laughter — sounds that transparently expressed how one felt in the moment. Ancient languages evolved out of those sounds. Gradually, words were formed to capture the essence of other things that helped form the matrix of life: the presences of trees, rocks, animals, and birds. In this sense, all ancient languages were originally mantric because their words embodied the essence of what they signified.

In Hinduism, mantric speech was considered especially sacred because it made present the reality of the thing signified by the sound. The Hebrew tradition reflects a similar awareness; one could not take the name of God in vain because the name of God summoned the presence of God — an overwhelming energy "too terrible to behold." Imagine how comfortably we use many powerful words today without connecting them to the depth or energy of what they signify. A famous passage from Patanjali's *Yoga Sutras* says: "The word *(shabda),* the object *(artha),* and the idea *(pratyaya)* appear as one [in ordinary discourse]; but by meditation *(samyama)* over their distinctions comes the knowledge of the sounds of all living beings."[4]

This "essential sound" of things is known as *Vak,* a feminine principle central to the Vedic tradition and revered as a Goddess. Vak represents "the speech of all things." Mantras, particularly Vedic mantras, are a form of "applied Vak." In the spiritual vision of Hindus, Vak is more sacred than ordinary speech and carries a far deeper significance. The Rishis are said to have visualized the mystic form of Vak, which is subtle, eternal, imperishable, and incomprehensible by ordinary sense organs.[5] The *Rg Veda,* the earliest of the four Vedas, states that three-quarters of the mysterious nature of Vak is hidden in heaven: "Vak was divided into four parts. These, those *Brahmans* [wise priests] with insight know. Three parts, which are hidden, mortals do not activate; only the fourth part they speak."[6]

The *Rg Veda,* composed entirely of mantric poems, is the earliest of the four Vedas. The other vedas are the *Sama Veda,* which are poems of the *Rg Veda* set to music; the *Yajur Veda,* comprised essentially of prose mantras and mantras associated with Vedic sacrifices; and the *Atharva Veda,* which deal with mantras of magic. Vak is essential to Shabda Yoga because it is central to the sacred speech of the Vedas, an underlying "language" of nature in which the sounds of cows, animals, birds, frogs, drums, and even inanimate objects participate because every sound, for those who are spiritually attuned, is a kind of speech.[7]

One of the first tasks of the postmodern sound yogi is to reconnect the words we use with the feelings associated with them. As language has evolved into its contemporary abstract form, we have learned to communicate without feeling — a disastrous condition for our relationships and our wholeness. Our present culture is based on the ability of human beings to communicate effectively with one another, but today we do so purely on an intellectual and technological level. We can, for instance, speak of God and not feel God; we can speak of love and be incapable of it; and, of course, we can speak of peace without truly desiring it. We have built our business infrastructures, our politics, our religion, and our personal relationships on words that can be said without feeling and still be understood.

Our task now is to rebuild our lives with words that fully embody the significance of their sounds. Once we reconnect our words with the experiences they signify, we bring the feminine back into our language and we reinstate the goddess Vak into our speech.

LEVELS OF SACRED SPEECH

THE VEDIC GRAMMARIANS differentiated among four levels of linguistic speech through which outer sound led to inner experience, and ultimately to Shabda Brahman, the absolute presence of the Divine Word. *Vaikari vak* is external speech, the dense outer sound of the "sounded word." *Madhyama vak* is the intermediate process of translating speech into understanding, as well as the reverse process of translating thoughts into speech. *Pasyanti vak* is unitive thought — the full comprehension of what is being communicated, invariably acknowledged by nodding in silence. In musical terminology, both speaker and listener are attuned to the same wavelength when the meaning of the words exchanged has been apprehended. If we could empathically sense what others were thinking and feeling, we wouldn't need words. While some Australian aboriginal tribes possess this ability, most of us can't communicate without the use of language.

But sacred speech goes even deeper, penetrating to a fourth level of *Para vak* — the great Word, the ultimate vibration in which the Divine dwells and thinks this universe into existence. Mantras are speech patterns that have the thrust and acceleration to find their way back to this primal level of speech because they originate at this deepest level. They are like guided mystical vehicles, programmed in their sonic nuance and meter to merge with Absolute Sound, the ultimate vibratory realm we've been referring to as Shabda Brahman.

These four levels of sacred speech —Vaikari, Madhyama, Pasyanti, and Para — are pivotal in using sacred sound as mantras and as a form of yoga. There are also four vibratory strengths for using mantras that correspond with these four levels of speech; I will introduce them at the end of this chapter. The path of sacred sound leads to enlightenment only when we follow the vibratory path of the mantra all the way into the depths of our consciousness, merging in samadhi with Shabda Brahman.

THE PROTECTION OF THE WORD

SHABDA YOGA teaches us to connect the dense, audible, outer word with inner meaning and experience. When we learn to do this effectively, we know where a person is coming from and to what end their words will take us. Such knowledge can protect us from those who don't mean well and help us differentiate between the authentic and the inauthentic. It also means that our own words will originate from a truth within us; when people connect with the vibration of words that come from such a depth, they too will be led to a truth within themselves.

Even in everyday use, we can recover the essence of words through conscious awareness of shabda in our normal exchanges. This requires that we carefully consider what we say and think, and that we stay attuned to the effects of our words on ourselves and others. The more we attune ourselves to the vibratory power of words, the more we will become inspired to methodically replace negative words and phrases with positive ones. Through this substitution, we affect ourselves emotionally by replacing fear with trust, hate with love, and anger with peace. This is the gift that a shabda yogi gives to the world, beginning within.

SOUND AND MEMORY

AS I MENTIONED, the Vedic seers understood Divine revelation to have two forms: sruti, meaning that which is heard, and smriti, that which is remembered. Vedic mantras, traditionally referred to as "sruti," are often recited aloud so that they are heard by the practitioner and can awaken the memory of protection and beneficence associated with the sounds. The vibrations of loud utterance are also for the benefit of the world, which absorbs them through a type of spiritual osmosis. Interestingly, the word "sruti" is also used to denote the fundamental tone in Indian music, which serves to help Indian musicians hear the pitch they are working in. In the same way, shabda mantras remind us that everything is being uttered by the Divine ground — the fundamental tone of all existence — and that we must stay connected to this Shabda Brahman, this absolute sound, this archetypal logos.

"Smriti," meaning "that which is remembered or recalled," traditionally refers to the sacred lore and laws that are passed on from generation to generation — ancestral wisdom, in other words. According to Vedic philosophy, shabda mantras should awaken the deep states of consciousness encountered by the Vedic Rishis because these mystical experiences are within our own memory. As long as we confine our study of mantras to reading "about" them, we are limited to the level of smriti, which is like the words of a story that help us remember an incident. Without having had the experience yourself, it is hard to relate to the story.

Sound, as shabda, should therefore be consciously employed in a manner that seeks to awaken us to the memory of our underlying cosmic consciousness — of our union with the Divine ground of being and all of creation. The following is a mantra from the Isa Upanishad that I like to use to collect my energies when I feel scattered or disempowered. The mantra translates as "Oh, my soul, remember everything good that you have strived for in the past, and recall this energy into the present moment."

Kra-to Sma-ra Kru-tam Sma-ra

SHABDA BRAHMAN: THE SONIC ABSOLUTE

BECAUSE SOUND and memory are so inextricably linked, sound can awaken us to the ultimate presence of God — a memory just waiting to be recalled. Our spiritual journey through time has been metaphorically described as a fall from primeval harmony and a forgetting of our true nature. Spiritual practice is meant to help us find our way back home — to the Om, so to speak. The role of sound in creation is underscored by the observations of John Cramer, a University of Washington physicist who developed an actual audio file of the "big bang," the sound origin of the universe, that can be played on your computer.[8] According to Dr. Cramer, the big bang wasn't an explosive sound at all, but more like a deep hum, which is exactly what the Rishis perceived in their meditations and uttered as Om.

Shabda Yoga should therefore be practiced with the intention of awakening ourselves to our highest potential, our deepest spiritual identity, and our Divine ancestry. Just as we can discover the true meaning and essence behind the words of everyday human existence, the practice of Shabda Yoga can awaken us to the memory of the Divine Presence, stored inside us and waiting to break through. When this happens, we see all things as emanations from a common source that awaken in us the words of St. Thomas Aquinas: that we, indeed, are a word of God. The universe then becomes a "web of interdependent and interconnected relationships," a phrase made popular by physicist Fritjof Capra in his work, *The Tao of Physics*.[9]

CREATING HARMONY AND ORDER

IN CHAPTER THREE, we discussed "rta," the Vedic sense of order and harmony that pervades the universe and creates a basic drive toward harmony in all living creatures. Even with those aspects of the physical world that we consider to be inanimate — without life, without breath — we can perceive order, structure, and harmony in their symmetry and molecular construction. Another clear sign that our own being is vibrating in sympathy with cosmic consonance is the fact that, no matter how much we deviate into disharmony, we feel at peace when harmony is restored.

The harmony that pervades our universe was intuited by early Greek philosophers such as Pythagoras and Ptolemy, and later proved by Johannes Kepler in the seventeenth century through his *Music of the Spheres.* Today, scientists say that music is ubiquitous in nature (the earth herself hums a tune), and that musical harmony shows up in the arrangements of the planets, in seascapes, and even in our brain waves.[10] Robert Roy Britt, a science writer for *Space.com,* writes: "A CD of black-hole music most likely can't compete with Britney Spears or the Soggy Bottom Boys, but a new study shows these venerable gravity instruments produce complex tunes whose underlying principles are remarkably similar to pop, bluegrass, classical, or any other style you might think of."[11]

The evidence is in. Our motivation is to now trust in the harmony of the universe and allow this harmony to influence our thoughts, our words, and our emotions. This means that we consciously make use of ancient and sacred languages that embody this harmony in our spiritual and yoga practice. The practice of Shabda Yoga, through the recitation of Vedic mantras in Sanskrit, can help us achieve this sense of cosmic order by organizing the energy in our lives into structured and harmonic form, transforming life into music and speech into poetry.

APPLIED COSMOLOGY

When we discover the mantric power of sound, we learn to live in a cosmic context; we feel that we belong to the universe. The concept of the "university," a term coined in the Middle Ages by European monks, was of a center where people would learn to find their place in the universe, helping them discern their role in the grand scheme of things and play their part in a great symphony. Ours is an amazingly sonorous universe. From DNA and the atomic structure of oxygen to the blossoming of a rose and the hum of planets, we encounter sounds as familiar as the music of Bach. Indeed, Willie Ruff and John Rogers of Yale University created music by programming the angular velocities of the planets into a synthesizer, precisely following the mathematical equation of Johannes Kepler. Joachim-Ernst Berendt says the following about their resulting recording:

> *Mercury, the fast and restless "messenger of the gods," does indeed have a quick, busy, chirping, "quicksilvery" sound. Aggressively and ruthlessly, Mars slides up and down across several notes. Jupiter has a majestic tone reminiscent of a church organ, and Saturn produces a low, mysterious droning.*[12]

Recovering our sense of cosmology is imperative. Isolating ourselves more and more in our automobiles and high-rise buildings, we estrange ourselves from the earth, the stars, and the heavens. Shabda Yoga is applied cosmology; it lets us rediscover, directly and immediately, that we are each like little universes, part and parcel of an immense cosmos made up of innumerable universes like ourselves. This immensity moves us beyond the limits of the ego, enabling us to embrace a Self that is magnanimous. We become great souls in the process, for that is what the word means: *magna* meaning "great," and *animus* meaning "soul."

A POSTURING OF THE SOUL

Shabda Yoga, because of its complex consonants, poetic nuance, and grammatical syntax, sculpts and shapes the energies of our soul in a special way. It offers protection from negative forces and configures our energy to attract beneficial circumstances into our lives. To use words and sounds in this consciously sacred manner is to posture the soul — in much the same way that Hatha Yoga, through its postures, sculpts and shapes the slower or denser energies of the body. Proper posturing of the soul enables us to feel better, think better, and act better.

To enter into a day-to-day experience of Shabda Yoga, we must learn to use our speaking and thinking language for spiritual purposes. We do this by reconnecting feeling and experience to the words we use in our private lives, in our homes, in our relationships, and in our professional environments. In addition, we must simultaneously develop a sacred language for the needs of our soul. As with all mantras, I highly recommend Sanskrit for this purpose, but you may choose otherwise if your ancestral roots resonate more strongly with another tongue.

In Hatha Yoga, postures (asanas) and stretches create a strong, balanced infrastructure that helps optimally channel and distribute energies generated by breath practices, or pranayama. In the same way, posturing the soul through the sounds of Shabda Yoga allows us to introduce bija mantras, or the energetic seed syllables characteristic of Shakti Yoga, the stream of sacred sound that we will explore in the next chapter.

A SIMPLE EXERCISE IN SHABDA YOGA

THIS EXERCISE will help you experience the power of Shabda Yoga in relation to familiar words and concepts. The Sanskrit term is associated with the specific vibratory consistency of each type of utterance. Think of something you want very much and encode this need in a short phrase, such as, "I want to feel ___________." Then use the following steps to work with your desire:

1. *Vachaka:* Get in touch with your emotions, and articulate what you feel clearly and confidently by saying your phrase aloud three times to activate the dense, physical form of the physical-material plane and have it conform to your statement.
2. *Upaamsu:* Soften the sound by whispering it three times into the air. This brings the message to the emotional-energetic plane and strengthens the power of your statement. As you take your words to this subtler layer of being, you will feel

closer to your heart space. Sounding in this manner helps you release your fears and doubts.

3. *Maanasa:* Say the phrase three times in your mind, slowly, clearly, and confidently. You are now affecting the deep substructures of your being and reconfiguring your core belief system to accommodate what you are speaking, thus activating the causal-spiritual plane of our existence.
4. *Tusnim:* Become internally quiet and just listen. When you listen with your whole body, you will feel the effects of your Shabda Yoga practice. It is as though your soul were speaking in silence to the Divine, who is listening in silence.

While it is possible to feel the effects of this exercise using ordinary words, imagine what could happen if you were to employ actual Sanskrit mantras. Try the method again, this time using a prayer phrase, such as *Om Namah Christaaya, Shivaaya Namah Om,* a sacred word such as *Shanti* (peace), or even your core mantra. Notice how quickly you can feel the power of the words you are uttering and how effectively you can journey into the heart.

Traditional Vedic mantras, as you will see in appendix one, are complex mantric phrases designed to illuminate, protect us, and draw beneficial circumstances into our lives. They are usually chanted just once, or possibly three times.

Remember that the external sound is always paramount in Shabda Yoga. To feel the progressive vibratory experience of any type of mantra, chant it nine times: thrice audibly, thrice softer on the breath (in a whisper), and thrice internally in your mind. These three variations also correspond with three planes of existence: the physical-material plane, the subtle-energetic plane, and the causal-spiritual plane. You want to reach a state in which you can say a word or phrase just once and recognize the complete experience of feeling that goes along with the idea or thought that the word signifies.

The method we are using makes us consciously aware of the progressive movement of all linguistic processes, from vaikari through madhyama to pasyanti, retracing sound's manifestation in the physical world, through our emotional field, to the causal level of spirit. Gradually, with

Divine grace, we can break through to the great Sound, the great Word — Para Vak — and encounter Shabda Brahman, the vibratory presence of the Divine itself.

THE MUSIC OF SHABDA YOGA

VEDIC MANTRAS are often chanted using just three tones. A fundamental tone, which I call the base tone, is the default pitch; it should be centered in the heart. By this I mean that you should choose a comfortable tone that resonates in your mid-chest. A high tone is to be used above the base tone, and a low tone below it; this causes the energy of the mantra to move into the head and belly, alternating between these three essential centers of reference. This pattern of chanting is common in Jewish cantor and in the tones of liturgical prayer in Catholic or Episcopalian masses.

Although it is possible to speak many traditional Vedic mantras, the use of tones confers a special quality. Certain Vedic mantras, such as the *Rudram* of the *Yajur Veda,* must be chanted because the Rishis perceived certain specific tones and prescribed them for yogic transformation.

For those of you who are musically adept, I recommend that you use a half-tone above your fundamental base tone for your morning practice and a whole tone above the base tone for evening practice. This matches the energy of those times of the day. For the tone below the base tone, a whole tone is appropriate for both morning as well as evening recitation of Vedic mantras.

Comparing the Vedic mantras on the accompanying audio tracks with those in appendix one will help you distinguish between the half-tone and whole-tone variation. More information about tones and musical intervals is provided in chapter ten, "Nada Yoga."

In appendix one, you will see Vedic mantras positioned along three lines so that you can gauge how the mantra moves among the three tones. Even if you don't feel musically knowledgeable and need to approximate, moving among these tones will optimally calibrate the flow of your mental energies.

During Vedic rituals and ceremonies, Shabda Yoga mantras can go on continuously for days, recited by groups of Brahmin* priests

---

* To clarify these terms, a *Brahmin* is a Vedic priest; *Brahman* is ultimate reality; and *Brahma* is God the Creator.

who alternate their breath cycles so that no pause occurs in the complex recitations of the set formulae. Because the tones are prescribed by scripture, the priests can come in precisely with phonetic accuracy.

The power of moving among three tones sustains the wavelength of sound frequencies generated by our brain, streamlining our mental processes toward the intention of the mantra. This is dhyana, the seventh limb of Raja Yoga, which leads to samadhi. The brain waves of consciousness are discussed in chapter sixteen.

In closing, I'd like to suggest that you regularly channel your practice of Shabda Yoga into the tones of everyday speech. Take care to use kind and gentle tones as much as possible; at other times, be firm yet loving. In *The Mozart Effect,* Don Campbell quotes the outgoing message of a little girl on her mother's answering machine: "After the beep, please leave your tone."[13] The vibratory effects of our tones, in both speech and written communications, find their way deep into the psyche — our own as well as that of the person who receives the message. Let us be mindful about these tones and use our voices to heal rather than to hurt.

CHAPTER 8

SHAKTI YOGA:
RENEWING ENERGY THROUGH TANTRIC MANTRAS

Shakti Yoga is the path of energy. In this stream of Sound Yoga, the expansive resonance of the word — shabda — is brought home to the human body in the form of shakti mantras. These sounds are Tantric, or rooted in the body, whereas Vedic mantras are oriented toward the cosmos. We could say that, in the Tantric tradition, mantras incarnate as flesh and blood, emphasizing the immanence of the Divine presence rather than the transcendence evoked by the poetry of Vedic mantras.

"Tantra" means "fabric," and refers to the warp-and-woof intermeshing of life and consciousness. The roots of Tantrism lie in closely guarded esoteric insights from the pre-Vedic tradition of goddess worship, which coexisted with, intermingled with, and influenced the Vedic period. It then experienced a resurgence around 500 A.D. with the development of many key Tantric texts.

In the Tantric view, the feminine energy of Shakti is considered to be the agent of all Divine action. With beautiful philosophical balance, every male deity in the Hindu tradition has a corresponding *shakti* — a female counterpart. In Hinduism, the feminine shakti is perceived as the *active* principle, which is a reversal of the Western view. Shakti, for the Hindu, is a dynamic energy without which nothing can be accomplished. Shiva, the pervasive male principle, is thus complemented by Shakti, the pervasive female principle. Similarly, Brahma the Creator is complemented by Saraswati, the goddess of art and knowledge, and Vishnu the preserver is balanced with Lakshmi, the goddess of wealth and abundance. All goddesses are forms of the one shakti. The absolute sound, Shabda Brahman, is complemented by the absolute energy, *Para Shakti.* It should be noted, however, that at the level of Brahman, or supreme reality, gender is subsumed and transcended. Here reality is viewed through the single eye — the eye of wisdom between the eyebrows — while all other views of reality are through the eyes of duality. Tantrics see the play of opposites in all aspects of creation as contributing to dualistic modes of perception, which must be unified, embodied, and transformed through the process of Tantric Yoga.

BLOOD OF THE GODDESS

In Tantric mysticism, the throbbing at the heart of all creation is called *spanda*. This primal humming of the Divine presence is a tremendous bidirectional vortex of power, intelligence, and energy, spinning constantly and effortlessly while generating the multitude of sound vibrations that become the universe. Information continually flows outward to every aspect of creation and is simultaneously received from every facet of being through an eternal process that composes the music of life. This sounds a lot like Candace Pert's "molecules of emotion," as mentioned in chapter one, but in this case it's occurring on a macroscopic level.

Shakti is the raw energy that gushes out of spanda, coursing excitedly through all vibrations and endowing them with life and vitality. She is the blood of the universe, rushing in and out of its deep center, purifying and renewing all that has become contaminated. Shakti is like the human heart, receiving impure blood through the veins and sending purified blood to every part of the body through the arteries. Two of Shakti's infinite faces demonstrate that this inescapable energy is fierce as well as loving, capable of creation as well as destruction: *Kali* is a dark being who receives the impure wastes generated by the creative process, while *Durga* is a being of light who confers grace and blessing upon all.

Out of context, Kali and Durga are feared for their fierce symbolism and terrifying forms — Kali with her necklace of skulls, and Durga riding her powerful tiger. But only our ego fears them, with its desire to fragment reality and "cut the fabric of life" to its own tastes and desires. When the ego is surrendered, we become free to love and to accept change. We become part of a great cosmic design. If we hold fast to our conditioned reflexes and live purely from our head, we may one day find ourselves decapitated, our skull strung on Kali's necklace. We cannot fight wholeness for long. One day, life will turn and we will be forced to surrender our center of reference.

On the opposite end of the spectrum from Kali, Durga's tiger represents animal instinct under the benign influence of the wise goddess who rides it. Riding the tiger also has a sexual connotation of benign energy channeled toward its own source in the sexual act. Once we surrender to the source, we discover that our center — whether previously located in the mind or in the genitals — is present everywhere. Christian mystic and scientist Nicholas of Cusa once described the Divine as a circle, with its center everywhere and its circumference nowhere. This is what we discover through the Tantric process.

THE BODY: A MICROCOSM OF THE UNIVERSE

As we advance through stages of spiritual evolution, we discover various centers and forms of energy through our sexuality, our individuality, our capacity to relate lovingly, our creativity, and our power to think and examine. Sometimes people get stuck at one stage, as when someone becomes obsessed by sexuality or when one lives completely in the rational mind, cynical about everything and disconnected from emotion. Shakti Yoga shows us how we can bring together these various forms of energy and orchestrate these differentiated planes of existence into harmonious balance and wholeness. In other words, we must eventually learn to live from our deepest center — not from our head, gut, genitals, or sentiments, but from the very bottom of our soul. It is undeniably the heart that offers us the greatest amount of fulfillment, and life is always pushing us to realize this essential truth.

Movement is an essential aspect of Shakti Yoga. We want to move *through* our centers of reference in the head, the gut, and our sexual organs and allow ourselves to find our way into the very heart of all existence. In Shakti Yoga, the physical body incarnates the energy of the soul; it is a conduit for all the information life has to offer, and it functions as a vehicle for the soul. Christian mystic St. Gregory Palamas once wrote, "The body, too, is capable of divine things when the passionate forces of the soul are not put to death, but transformed and sanctified."[1] This is exactly what we must discover today.

Basic physics teaches us that form is energy and energy is form. This is why the mantras and practices of Shakti Yoga can be used to direct the flow of energy in and through the body. As shown by Hans Jenny's experiments in cymatics, described in chapter one, various substances — sand, spores, iron filings, water — organize themselves in harmonic patterns when exposed to specific sounds, such as live or recorded music, or human vocalization.[2] Solid objects, as we know, are composed of comparatively slow-moving molecules. Their vibratory structure is more compact and thus less permeable. Liquid, on the other hand, is more fluid, but it is still subject to the force of gravity; these molecules are less compacted. Gases are airy, free, expanded, and made up of extremely fast-moving molecules. Having a "sound" physical body means having optimal flow and consistency of energy in our solid, liquid, and gaseous structures. Our blood flow should be free and unobstructed, air should enter our lungs unimpeded, pure body fat must be properly contained, and our muscles should be well toned. Shakti mantras, like musical tones, can aid this process by dissolving constricted energy blocks, improving the flow of energy in all its varying consistencies. These mantras operate on the same principle as the lithotripter, which dissolves kidney stones, or as the opera singer who can shatter a crystal goblet. We can see how sound and music can contribute significantly to improved health.

BALANCING MASCULINE AND FEMININE ENERGIES

Tantra assigns human sexuality a central place in the spiritual process. The sexual center of the human body is seen as a storehouse of power — a reservoir from which we can channel energy toward other centers in the body. In Shakti Yoga, the channels that conduct the flow of energy are known as *nadis.* Nadis constitute a system that is somewhat similar to the meridian system of Chinese acupuncture, but based on a subtler plane of existence. The energy conducted through these channels is known as *prana.* Prana is the vital life force present in all things; it is conducted into living organisms through the medium of air — the same medium through which sound waves travel.

The nadis are a subtle network comprised of seventy-two thousand channels, three of which are the most important. The main channel, called the *susumna,* is located alongside the spinal cord and runs all the way from the base of the spine to the crown of the head. When energy is directed into this channel, the highest spiritual goals can be realized. But the human body, in Tantric practice, is also divided in two equal halves. On either side of the central susumna are two important sub-channels, known as *ida* and *pingala.* Ida, associated with the left side of the body, is linked to lunar energy; it is both feminine and cooling by nature. Pingala is associated with masculine energy and solar power; it is by nature hot, and linked to the right side of the body.

Each channel is also associated with a specific hemisphere of the brain and is governed by a specific nostril. Ida, the feminine channel, originates from the left side of the spinal base, culminates in the left nostril, and governs the right hemisphere of the brain. Pingala, which governs the left hemisphere of the brain, originates toward the right of the spinal base and culminates in the right nostril. Activities requiring physical strength and dexterity draw energy from the right, masculine nostril, while those requiring emotional strength draw from the left. To realize spiritual objectives in yoga, both energies must be unified and simultaneously directed up the central susumna through all the *chakras* — the seven vortexes of power that govern our emotional, mental, and spiritual states.

Long ago, yogis noticed that the right, or solar, nostril dominates during the day, while the left, or lunar, nostril dominates at night. This natural process allows for vigorous activity during the daytime and leisure and sleep at night. One can deliberately alter these patterns for specific explorations in energy and consciousness through *Swara Yoga,* a branch of yoga that specializes in nostril control. "Swara" means "that which makes its own sweetness." It is also the word used for musical notes — do, re, mi, and so on. We can discern here a direct correlation among sound, breath, emotional states, and the chakras. In chapter thirteen, you will learn how Western medical doctors listen to the sound and music of the breath to understand the health status of our body.

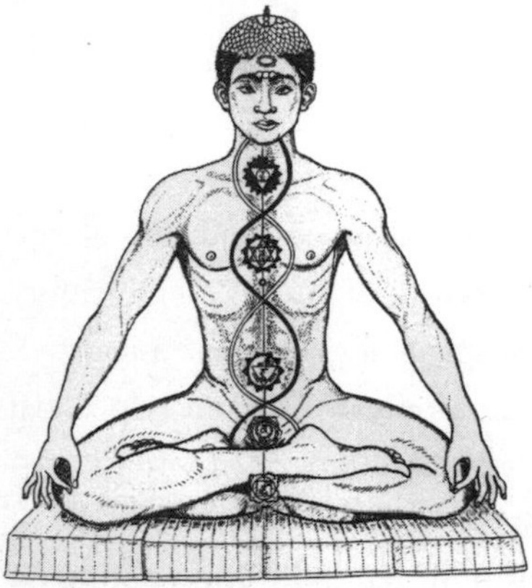

Ida and pingala intertwine around the chakras to create a helix-like pattern similar to the caduceus, a winged staff entwined by two serpents that symbolizes healing in Western medicine. These serpents are symbols of the Greek and Roman gods Hermes and Mercury. In a bit of cross-cultural symmetry, the serpent symbolizes consciousness in the East. As East continues to meet West on so many levels, we can see the connection between healing and consciousness growing deeper with time.

CHAKRAS: PLAYING THE MUSIC OF THE SOUL

THE CHAKRAS are hubs that allow energy to pass through them and become transmuted into experiences. Along the spine are five human chakras, or vortexes; entry and exit vortexes at either end of the spine bring the total to seven. Among the five human vortexes, the genitals are the storehouse for primal energy; the power to organize and govern lies in the abdomen; the capacity to love is located in the heart; the throat holds the passage of creativity and imagination; and in the center of the forehead is the seat of wisdom and inner perception.

At the base of the spine, close to the anal opening, is the "root support" or *muladhara* chakra, through which we interface with raw, undifferentiated energy. Through this threshold, primal shakti energy enters the body. This unbridled power then makes itself present in the body, first and foremost as our sex drive — which my mentor Bede Griffiths often described as the fundamental love instinct in human nature.

The crown of the head, or "crown chakra," is the exit point for energy. After being transmuted through all our chakras, our basic life force can here be transformed into blissful Divine energy. This is the goal of Shakti Yoga, or Tantra Yoga.

The word "chakra" means "wheel" or "discus," indicating the dynamic, spinning motion of these centers. Today, the analogy of a spinning CD or DVD metaphorically describes how these centers hold tremendous amounts of information. Physiologically, medical experts have identified complex crossovers of nerves and glandular secretions that can be directly associated with each of the chakras and the energies they govern. All of our experiences are stored in the chakras: sexual experiences are held in the sexual chakra; romantic and filial experiences in the heart; creative experiences in the throat center. Experiences are constantly awakened and relived when energy is activated in the chakras, giving rise to the distinct states of consciousness related to various types of energy — sexual, emotional, mental — that we experience in everyday life. Chakras, in other words, play the music of our soul.

Opening the Chakras

When energy flow is unimpeded in our body, it travels effortlessly through the chakras and carries with it all our experiences, which find ultimate fulfillment when merged with the Divine Presence. But the natural journey of our energy from the base of the spine to the top of the head is often blocked. Unresolved experiences restrict the passage of energy through a particular chakra. Resolved experiences pose no obstruction; they actually configure the chakra to allow energy to pass through it.

Creative, artistic people are often open and vulnerable, but they can also be blocked in the abdomen and intimidated by organizational demands. Intellectuals can be brilliant thinkers but incapable of getting in touch with their emotions. Sexually obsessive individuals may have poor control over their emotions, and excessively loving people can be overwhelming if their love is not balanced with perspective. This is all because it is possible for us to operate from a dominant chakra, while being constricted in others. Complete blockage will result in disease, or even death. But constriction, irregular flow, or misdirection of energy is not uncommon in the chakras we are unwilling to open and heal.

As we live and act in the world — especially a busy one — we build up resistance in an effort to defend ourselves. But resistance prevents flow, and the lack of flow creates discomfort — which, if not attended to, eventually leads to disease. The trauma of being physically attacked, for instance, or even a hurtful conversation may become stored as blockage in our body and our chakras. As a consequence, we might create the habit of tightening our belly or unconsciously constricting our heart space. These are like scratches on a record. Shakti Yoga shows us how to get the needle out of the repetitive groove and let new music play.

Psychology is a powerful tool because it helps us dissolve the blockage in our chakras. Some psychologists, including Jungian analyst Ashok Bedi, M.D., are using Shakti Yoga techniques in their psychotherapy practices to assist in releasing blocked energy. In his book *Path to the Soul,* Dr. Bedi uses the seven-chakra system of Shakti Yoga to describe how the soul sends out emergency signals from the depths of the psyche.[3] And some medical doctors, notably Dharma Singh Khalsa, M.D., are using the age-old practices of Shakti Yoga in their treatments of physical ailments with tremendous success. Such practices are no doubt rare, but the stage is being set for an integrative medicine that employs yogic practices and insights in the healing process because the body and the soul are indivisible in the realm of spirit.

ENERGY'S DESTINATION: ENLIGHTENMENT

The mantras of Shakti Yoga gently and methodically work on our obstructions by releasing healing energy in the chakras, which then open up to the flow. This is why chakras are often depicted in esoteric Hindu art as flowers with opening petals. When primal energy is allowed to pass through all the chakras without obstruction, its merging with the Divine Presence creates an intense light that causes each chakra to turn upward and receive its warmth. This is exactly what happens in an awakened or enlightened soul — a *jivan mukta* — who has learned to channel, release, and merge personal energy with the Divine Absolute.

Classical and religious art — particularly Christian art — often depicts saintly people with halos around their heads. This representation is more than metaphorical. It is, in fact, an accurate insight into the merging of our individual consciousness with the Divine Presence. Achieving a powerful, unobstructed flow of energy from the base of the spine to the top of the head and out through the crown indicates a profound union between body, soul, and spirit. This is samadhi, and sages from every culture have borne witness to the joy of this ecstatic union.

Somewhere deep within us, we know that our energy does indeed have a destination, and that its innate intelligence can guide it toward that goal if only we can learn to stay out of its way. There is, therefore, a devotional aspect of Shakti Yoga that asks for the grace of the mother, as Para Shakti (Supreme Energy) or Kundalini Maatha (Mother Kundalini), to dissolve our ego, rendering it transparent so that energy may pass through all the chakras effortlessly. The actual methodology of this devotion is addressed in the next chapter, "Bhava Yoga."

YANTRAS

Yantras are geometric cosmological diagrams that are created from special materials and embedded with mantras to produce specific conditions and transformations. The preparation of yantras involves strict rules of fasting and ritual actions that must be performed according to Tantric mantra-shastra. Each feminine deity in the Tantric tradition has her own cosmological diagram, which is carefully constructed using metals that conduct the energies associated with that particular goddess. For example, the Divine force of Shakti is electromagnetic, so copper, with its power to optimally conduct electricity, is a common choice for Shakti yantras. The Sanskrit letters of mantras are written or embossed into the completed yantra, which can then be hung either inside or outside the home

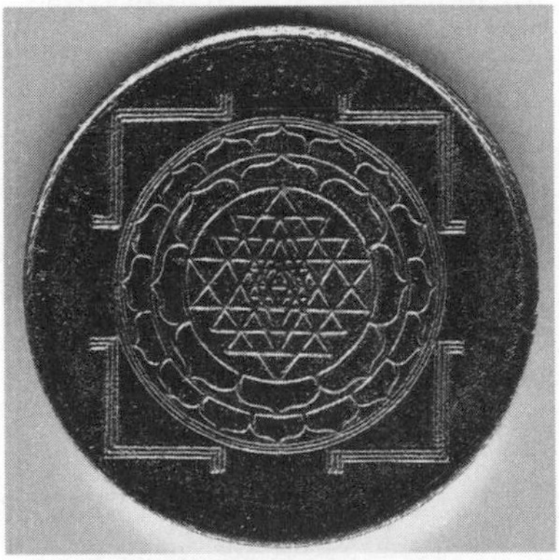

The Shree Yantra, associated with the goddess Lakshmi

or office to affect a person's life and relationships. If you are visually oriented and wish to learn to construct yantras that can be beneficial to your mantra practice, see Harish Johari's book *Tools for Tantra*.[4]

TRANSFORMING THE BODY THROUGH SOUND

The Tantric belief is that mantras, because of their potent power of encoding catalytic energy, can effect transformation by themselves; yet ritual is vital to Tantrism, as it provides the practitioner with a meaningful way to respect, embody, and develop a relationship with pure energy. Tantric rituals therefore often involve mystical gestures and actions that are performed along with mantras. An example is the *Sandhya Upaasana* ritual at the end of appendix one. As I mentioned, the Vedic tradition was strongly influenced by the Tantric tradition and incorporated many of its practices and methods. However, Vedic practitioners sought to keep the wildness of Tantricism under institutional control. Many Tantric rituals involve similar purification processes, performed by touching body parts while reciting mantras or even the Sanskrit alphabet. This identifies every part of the body with the rest of the universe, transforming the worshipper's body into the cosmos. A variation of this process is called *Anga-nyaasa,* a series of reverential mantras offered to parts of the body to consecrate them as being implicitly identical to those of the Supreme Deity. A typical version is the following, from the *Maha Nirvana Tantra,* one of the classic scriptures of Tantrism. Try touching the parts of your body named in parentheses as you pronounce these mantras.

Hraam Namaha (to the heart)
Hreem Svaaha (to the head)
Hruum Vausat (to the crown-lock)
Hraim Hoom (to the upper arms)
Hraum Vausat (to the three eyes: two out-seeing,
and the third unified)
Hraah Phat (to the two palms)[5]

The power of these mantras to transform consciousness is palpable only when you have built a strong practice of Sound Yoga. Pronouncing these mantras out of context can only hint at their power, or may even seem meaningless to the uninitiated.

A PHARMACY OF THE SOUL

As you will find in appendix one, many Shabda Yoga mantras, with the exception of the *Gayatri,* are repeated only three times. Some Shabda Yoga mantras, such as the *vyaahritis,* constitute a series that is recited just once each in sequence. Shakti Yoga mantras, on the other hand, emphasize repetition and are usually simpler in form and construction. Most often, the same sound is repeated many times to facilitate and intensify the healing energy in a specific area. Also, Shakti mantras generally do not use musical intervals; they are simply pronounced without any attempt to beautify them, uttered in raw simplicity using the natural voice, channeling energy without affectation. The only dynamic variable in the Shakti mantra recitation is the intensity of the utterance, which matches the natural intensity of the exhaled breath. Unlike Vedic mantras, Tantric mantras are most powerful when chanted internally or whispered softly on the breath.

Shakti mantras are also known as "bija mantras," meaning "seed syllables," since these primal sounds encase energy much like a capsule produced by a pharmaceutical company contains healing chemicals or herbs. While the Rishis and grammarians of the Vedic tradition emphasized dhvani, the audible word, and sphota, the illumination awakened by the referred experience of the word, the Munis of the Tantric tradition maintained an external silence by vowing not to speak. Instead, they directed their sonic experience deep into the physiology of the human body, focusing intently on internal repetition (maanasa). Like cosmic pharmacists, they took the energy that manifests in the thunder and lightning and plants and bees and ocean currents, and found a way to represent it in mantra capsules.

In order to ensure that the disposition of the ego does not diminish their efficacy, bija mantras associated with deities are often encased in a devotional container of sacred sounds. For example, the mantra *Om Hoom Namaha* encases the core syllable *hoom,* which is a bija associated with Shiva. In this mantra, the sacred syllable *Om* and the reverent invocation *Namaha* soften the raw power of the mantra *hoom* by placing it within the context of personal devotion. *Namaha* means "I prostrate myself to you," "I offer you my respect," or "I surrender." Several of these deity bijas are listed in appendix two, and an example of the encased form is also provided on the accompanying audio tracks.

I like to think that the prefix and suffix of a mantra *(Om* and *Namaha)* hold the primal energy of that mantra in a sort of psychic gelatin capsule. The heat of our body and the passion of our spiritual practice dissolve the gelatin to release the healing power of the mantra in our soul. Think of how often we imbibe medication without offering our respect to the healing energy contained in it; we take for granted that the medicine will do its work. Tantrism teaches us to pay close attention to energy in all its forms and to respect the healing power of all substances, because energy is a vibration, it is a sound.

As mentioned, in Shakti Yoga practice the devotional sounds encasing a bija mantra also serve to soften the intensity of the mantra. I call it the "buffered" version of these powerful and therapeutic sounds. Without the devotional encasement, these mantras act at full strength.

Bija Mantras of the Chakras

The seed syllables, or bijas, used to facilitate the flow of energy in the three lower chakras are *lam, vam,* and *ram;* the three upper chakras are awakened by the sounds *yam, ham,* and *om.* (Please see appendix two for the pronunciation of these mantras.) The thousand-petaled lotus at the crown of the head has no sound; it is Shabda Brahman, the Sonic Absolute itself, and its mantra is the vibration of silence. The chakra bijas are to be used by themselves (without *Om* and *Namaha),* and are most effective with the hands positioned in *mudras (chin* or *gnana* mudra), as I will explain in the following section.

MUDRAS AND MANTRAS

Mudras, pronounced "moo-druhz," are specific mystical gestures of the hands that accompany the mantras. The thumb represents the Divine, while the index finger represents the human soul. In many yogic mudras, the thumb and index finger are joined, denoting the act of yogic union — the yoking of the individual to the cosmic. The other three fingers represent the *gunas,* or aspects of nature. The middle finger represents *sattwa guna,* or purity — the light principle. The ring finger represents *rajo-guna,* which is passion or the fire principle. The little finger represents *tamo-guna,* which is inertia or the darkness principle. These three fingers are held in harmonic balance so that the flux of the universe is equalized. For other associations, see page 256 in appendix two.

The two most common yogic mudras are *chin* mudra and *gnana* mudra. In both, the thumbs are in contact with the index fingers, while the remaining three fingers are held harmoniously in balance. Chin mudra is used for receptivity. The hands are placed on the thighs, with the palms held facing up, to channel energy from the base of the spine toward the crown of the head. Gnana mudra is used to ground our energy. The hands are placed on the knees, with the palms facing down so that the fingers facilitate the flow of energy downward from the crown of the head to the base of the spine.

In beginning Yoga of Sound practice, I recommend accompanying your mantras with only these two mudras. If you feel flighty or mentally distracted, use gnana mudra to help ground your energy in your body and in the earth. If you feel bogged down, drained of energy, or heavy in the stomach, use chin mudra to raise your energy and transform it into a subtler form. Several other mudras are described in appendix two.

THE BREATH OF LIFE

One important Shakti Yoga practice is the deep, full-cycle breath, otherwise known as the "complete yogic breath" (the particulars of which are detailed in chapter thirteen). The out-breath clears an unobstructed path along which energy can pass through the chakras, while the in-breath causes energy to be awakened at the base of the spine and conducted to the top of the head, breathing life and vitality into each chakra. This "refined" energy can then be drawn back into all the chakras.

The procedures of Shakti Yoga are very much like the process of refining oil. At the root chakra level, we are drilling deep into our system, causing primal energy to gush out and enter the sexual center. The Tantric yogi seeks to refine this primal energy through each of the chakras by producing various grades of activity in the vibration of the energy until it becomes the finest and purest form of Divine energy. This can be used to fuel the most sublime spiritual intentions and activities. Our first instinct is to release this energy on the sexual plane, which is why many Tantric practitioners require sexual experiences in the early stages of their practice; it helps them work off energy that cannot be contained. Over time, Tantrics learn to contain this energy and direct it upward, step by step, through each chakra until the energy can be emitted through the crown of the head. This achievement of merging all our experiences in Shabda Brahman brings with it the highest experience of samadhi, an unequaled ecstasy.

AWAKENING AND DIRECTING ENERGY

In the West, many workshops on Tantric practice promote awakening the primal Kundalini energy in the root chakra and channeling it into sexual activity and self-gratification. In the same way, Kundalini can be awakened in the root chakra and channeled into the abdominal area to dominate and control other people. Often, the first three chakras — root, sexual, and abdominal — are ruled by the ego, which makes our world a dangerous place.

The challenge of Shakti Yoga is to channel the energy, not just to these three lower chakras of physical and psychological power, but all the way into the three higher chakras of spiritual awakening. When energy is contained and progressively channeled upward, it can be allowed to penetrate the heart, the throat, and the forehead, transforming primal energy into love, creativity, and spiritual knowledge. Ultimate fulfillment occurs when our transformed energy merges with the Divine Presence at the crown of the head. This union is samadhi, a bliss that supercedes the range of human experience. When all seven chakras are activated and balanced, a deep flowering occurs.

Even if we don't consciously try to move energy into our chakras, the process occurs naturally all the time. Usually only small amounts of energy, or shakti, are being released into the body from the base of the spine. Yoga practice — especially Tantric Yoga or Kundalini Yoga, and also Hatha Yoga — seeks to intensify the flow of energy and prepare the nervous system to efficiently handle the increased intensity without causing a "brown-out" in our nervous system or short-circuiting our spiritual channels. The chakras exist to naturally condition the flow of primal energy in our body so that we can enjoy a variety of experiences — sexual, mental, creative, and so on. All these experiences are energetic in their essence, but most normal human experiences do not require that the flow of energy in the chakras be intensified. Only the advanced spiritual practitioner or Tantric yogi pushes the envelope to explore new horizons in the landscape of consciousness.

Yogis perceived that actions (karma) — especially repeated actions — create grooves *(samskaras)* in our chakras. If all we can think about is sex, that's where the energy goes. The result of this involuntary mechanism is that we keep investing our own shakti into a single chakra, or in looped patterns within several various chakras. Repeated patterns are the habits that we feed and reinforce, either consciously or unconsciously. Often, we are aware that certain mental, emotional, or behavioral patterns are unhealthy, but we are unable to effect the changes we desire; in the worst cases, we may even be completely unaware that change is needed in order for us to feel healthier.

The chanting of mantras is an effective way to clean our chakras, erase outmoded energy grooves, and encourage energy to flow in ways that offer a deeper perspective on life and a greater sense of purpose and meaning. In general, vowel sounds facilitate the flow of energy in and through the chakras, while consonants affect specific areas. When used repeatedly, consonants can strike the same region over and over again to disintegrate any obstruction to optimal energy flow.

Tantric experts agree with the advice of most financial experts: diversify your portfolio. This means regularly ensuring that energy doesn't accumulate in a single chakra for excessive periods of time because it can easily lead to burnout, disease, or the loss of valuable relationships. Once again, the use of vowel sounds and specific Shakti Yoga mantras can help distribute energy in the chakras and keep them operating efficiently. This will result in having more energy and more creative potential, with less stress and fewer negative emotions.

FINDING A UNIFIED APPROACH

Allowing shakti to flow up into the abdomen can give us great control of our emotions and excellent organizational capacity. Empowering this chakra helps remove fear and doubt. Many of us, rewarded by success in work, have obviously learned to do this effectively. When energy is directed farther upward, it enters the heart — something we often try to prevent, at least during business hours! Energy entering the heart becomes softer, like hard water being transformed in a water softener. When we become soft, we become vulnerable — and that's not good for business.

When shakti enters the heart, the ego melts and becomes transparent. We connect with our emotions and we begin to feel more deeply. Despite a capitalist system that rewards aggressive, analytical behavior, many of us work hard to be fully human in our work lives. It takes concerted effort to keep the energy flowing. We may fear compromising our career goals or becoming "too soft" if we're not aggressive. With all the pressure pointing us in that direction, we have to watch out for ego-acquisition modes that take over the chakras and make us less tolerant and compassionate.

By combining yogic streams in our community of mantras, we can achieve the necessary balance. When Shabda Yoga is employed in combination with Shakti Yoga, we become capable of making the soul vulnerable as well as strong, transparent as well as resilient. While seemingly paradoxical, this is not only possible but perhaps the only way to be fully human and still pursue our professional activities. Shabda Yoga offers us strength, protection, and a fortified emotional infrastructure that allows Shakti to enter the heart and pass on into the throat, where tremendous creative energy can be encountered. Today, we all have to wear many hats. In order to maintain inexhaustible creativity and a deep and fulfilling spiritual life, and simultaneously do well in our careers, we must learn to combine the streams of Sound Yoga into an effective daily practice. We will explore this in detail in part five of this book.

TANTRIC DEITY BIJA MANTRAS

The bija mantras may feel strange at first. Tantrism is rooted in the shamanic traditions of Hinduism and does, indeed, overlap with the magical, but there is no reason to fear them. Rather, we can revel in their exotic pleasures and feel them touch previously unexperienced parts of ourselves.

You may use bija mantras in their pure form for maximum potency, or you may place them between *Om* and *Namaha* for a time-release effect. For example, you might want to use *Om Hoom Namaha* or *Om*

Aim Namaha, a Saraswati bija. You may also combine the power of two mantras, for example *Om Hoom Aim Namaha.* Or you can repeat the same bija within a mantric phrase to emphasize a specific quality, for example, *Om Hoom Hoom Aim Shreem Namaha. Shreem* and *Shring* are bijas of Lakshmi, the goddess of wealth. See appendix two for more bija mantras and their energetic significance.

Shakti Yoga is about flow, so the use of movement is as important as the use of sound. Dancing the vowels, an exercise detailed in chapter fifteen, can be used with bija mantras to help open blocked energy in the chakras at any time of day.

JAPA: MANTRA REPETITION

The word *japa* means "repetitive prayer." As mentioned earlier, in the Tantric approach a mantra is repeated many times until the energy contained within the sound is released into the soul. The same process is used in the Jesus prayer, in which repeating the name of Jesus awakens in our heart a love for Jesus, drawing us into his presence. This is the teaching of the Christian Hesychast movement, a sort of Christian Tantrism that uses the pulse of the heart and the awareness of breath to stay centered in the body while repeating the name of Jesus. Monks of the Greek Orthodox Church on Mount Athos — the Mount Kailash of Christianity — developed this method of prayer.

In the Tantric tradition, the most powerful mantric repetition is in the depths of the heart. While the external sound is most important in Shabda Yoga recitation, Shakti Yoga emphasizes the internal sound. Internal recitation of mantras, as you will recall from the exercise at the end of chapter seven, is known as maanasa, "a sounding in the mind." In between loud vocalization and mental repetition, there is soft utterance or whispering, *upaamsu.*

MAALA: USING BEADS IN MANTRA RECITATION

Because the physical body is central to the experience of Tantrism, rosary beads are considered particularly helpful in the recitation of Shakti Yoga mantras. The beads also help with counting the number of recitations, another key element of Tantric practice, known as *purascharana.* Hindu yogic rosaries, called *maalas,* or *japa maalas,* usually have 108 beads, a number obtained by multiplying the number of planets in our solar system by the number of astrological signs in the zodiac. The number 108 originally represented the distances from the earth to the sun and the moon; both of these distances are approximately 108 times the respective diameters of the sun and moon.* You will recall from chapter two that, in Hatha Yoga, the syllable "ha" refers to the sun and "tha" to the moon, suggesting two opposite yet complementary energies that manifest in the body and the world. In Tantric Yoga, the sun and moon are associated with the ida and pingala nadis, which are the male and female channels on either side of the body. The use of maala beads balances our energies and allows the individual soul to be joined with the cosmos in yogic union. Our sonic meditation thus becomes a cosmological process that affects the entire universe.

One extra bead in the maala, known as *sumeru,* is never used because it represents Divine Presence itself. It is similar to the protection of the name of God in the Hebrew tradition or the avoidance of using an image of God in Islam. It shows the utmost reverence for the symbol directly identified with most high. We keep moving toward the sumeru as we recite our mantra; having arrived at our goal, we turn around and work our way toward it again from the other direction. The sumeru bead helps maintain a conscious awareness of ultimate Divine presence throughout the recitation. The process is the experience.

The materials from which a maala is made also have significance. Maalas made from rudraksha seeds are associated with Shiva's energy and are most often used by yogis, monks, and ascetics. Rudraksha maalas are excellent for developing detachment from worldly preoccupations and focusing on the eternal. The *tulasi* seed is associated with *Vishnu,* the preserver of the universe, and is used by householders and devotees of Krishna. Tulasi beads are used to preserve happiness in our relationships, both human and with the Divine. They are also used to generate peace and contentment within the family. Shakti worshippers use maalas made from turmeric, which is associated with

* The moon is 2,159 miles in diameter; multiply that by 108 and you get 233,000 miles, which is close to the distance between the earth and the moon (239,000 miles). The sun's diameter is 870,000 miles; multiply that by 108 and you get 93,960,000, which approximates the distance between the sun and the earth (93,000,000 miles).

fertility. Turmeric maalas are excellent for healing or for acquiring yogic powers. These maalas are biodegradable, and can therefore be buried in the ground or dissolved in a river after the desired result is achieved. Crystal is associated with Lakshmi, the goddess of wealth, and is therefore used to create affluence. Sandalwood, rosewood, and other types of maalas are also available. Generally, it is best to avoid synthetic materials.

Do not use the same maala for all your mantras. You can use your maala for your core mantra, or to achieve a specific goal using a specific mantra. If you change your core mantra, it is recommended that you use another maala, as the vibrations of another mantra would be different. This is not necessarily related to the type of maala; they could both be crystal, for instance. But a maala must be consecrated and dedicated for a particular mantra; the two must be exclusively partnered to infuse the maala with the power of the mantra.

After one hundred twenty-five thousand recitations of a mantra, the maala is considered independently empowered with shakti. The mantra, too, has reached its full potency for the practitioner at this time. In some cases, certain karmic factors may awaken the power of the mantra with a minimum of utterances. A person may have chanted this mantra many times in previous lives or simply have developed an open channel to its energy and vibrations. In such instances, the practitioner may simply breathe upon the maala to empower it with the shakti of the mantra. Once the maala has been charged with power, the beads used to recite it may be worn around the neck or placed on an afflicted area of a loved one for healing power and protection. A cotton string tied around the hand or foot may also be used in place of beads for this healing intention.

An important rule in maala recitation is that the index finger and little finger should not touch the beads. The beads are rolled between the middle finger and the thumb; the ring finger, not actively used, may contact the beads. This is a key teaching of mantra shastra. Other rules include facing east or north, considered the most desirable directions for recitation; proper diet; and the use of proper materials for the meditation seat. We shall discuss these practices further in chapter eleven.

LISTENING TO THE GODDESS

In chapter seven, we discussed Vak, which is personified as a goddess representing the speech of stones, water, animals, birds, insects, and humans. Vak is a principle shared by both Vedic and Tantric traditions. Meditation on Vak requires a deep listening to the birds, to the river, to the wind, to the thunder. To absorb the principle of Vak into our being is to embody the sacredness and vitality that pervade all of life. As we listen, we allow the power and essence of nature to be absorbed into our soul. This must be done without reflecting on the process. Vak is not to be understood; it is to be absorbed. A stone, a flower, a tree — even a house, a room, or a computer — is alive with energy and presence. These sounds can feed energy into our soul if we open our hearts to their presence. Meditation on Vak teaches us to move out of our self-preoccupied worlds and engage in the vibratory presence of things; the world is alive and throbbing with energy and intelligence.

Following the Goddess Home

You will remember that, in Shabda Yoga, sacred speech is perceived as unfolding in four phases, a process that recedes back into itself just like the universe. Emerging from the source, Shabda Brahman — the Sonic Absolute — has a thought (pasyanti). Through a magical process we call "nature" (represented by the term *madhyama,* or "middle process in speech") the thought translates into a flower or an elephant. We attune ourselves to this middle process in speech by the whispered breath in mantra practice; the manifest elephant or flower corresponds to the audible word, vaikari. To put it plainly, the Divine thought becomes a physical form by means of the Divine breath.

In Tantric mantra repetition, we use this understanding to reverse the process, using our own breath to move from an awareness of the physical plane to the Divine essence and energy. Thus, the outermost form of pronouncing the mantra (vacaka) moves into whispering the mantra on our breath (upaamsu), which then leads to sounding the mantra internally in our mind (maanasa). The deepest presence of sound, word, and mantra is actually a listening with all of our being, *tusnim,* the direct attunement to Shabda Brahman at the level of Para Vak or Supreme

Word. This happens when we are no longer saying the mantra, but the mantra is saying itself in us.

We therefore use the external sound to get the dense aspects of our being — cells, bones, tissues, and vital organs — to reverberate with the resonance of the mantra. Gradually we progress inward, through distinctly subtler levels, until we arrive at Para Vak or Shabda Brahman, the source of all sound and the ground of all being. As we try to penetrate all these levels of speech and sound, we must navigate through the resistance of our analytical mind. We may experience moments when we don't feel connected to the sacred. Often the analytical mind accompanies our efforts all the way to the source level, and it is only in that deep space that it eventually relinquishes all its tricks and habitual patterns. Single-minded determination is therefore required to follow the path of the mantra all the way home.

When we follow the vibration of the mantra all the way to its depth in Para Vak, we "follow the goddess home" — even if we don't sense her encouragement along the way. In other words, we must have faith that Divine grace is always with us as we use the mantra to navigate the dark alleyways of the mind. Obviously, this is not a principle we should employ for the wrong reasons, such as pursuing a process toward self-gratification, but for spiritual realization and the transformation of consciousness — the genuine objectives of Shakti Yoga.

CHAPTER 9

BHAVA YOGA:
FINDING ECSTASY THROUGH BHAKTI MANTRAS

Bhava is sheer ecstasy, a condition caused when the heart is seized by the Divine embrace. In Bhava Yoga, the cosmic power of Brahman in the Vedas — awakened through the complex mantras of Shabda Yoga as well as the mysterious, often unintelligible bijas of the Tantric tradition — becomes more approachable through devotion. "Bhava Yoga" is the term I prefer to use for the sonic stream of devotion found within the Bhakti tradition of Hinduism. "Bhakti" means devotion, while "bhava" is the state of mind or consciousness associated with devotion. The term "Bhava Yoga" helps us differentiate sacred sound used as a yoga path toward devotional ecstasy from the sacred words used for strength and protection in Shabda Yoga or the mystic syllables used for energy in Shakti Yoga.

The Bhakti tradition officially began between the first and second century B.C., although its existence precedes that era by about a thousand years. The *Bhagavad Gita,* dated around 600 B.C., emphasizes devotion — Bhakti Yoga — among the many paths of yoga. Bhakti started to become a powerful movement around 800 A.D., reached its peak in the Middle Ages, and was firmly established by 1700 A.D. Its popularity may have been a reaction to Shabda Yoga's strict rules of grammar and pronunciation on one hand, and the Tantric schools' secrecy and rigorous asceticism on the other. An interesting parallel was the oppressive regime of Muslim rule in India (711–1775 A.D.) and the destruction and desecration of many ancient and sacred Hindu temples during that period. These extremities may have propelled this movement of devotional chanting and singing into existence.

The accessible spirit of bhakti allows a less technical approach to sacred sound, drawing worship into the simplicity of the human heart without the complex hierarchies of spiritual systems. This was a significant development in the Yoga of Sound, as it invited the ordinary householder to practice mantras with freedom and confidence. Through the use of simple melodies, the devotional and musical chanting of mantras became a powerful way of finding union with the Beloved in whatever form of Divinity one felt drawn to.

Bhava points to the state of "being in the heart" that devotional mantras evoke; this state of samadhi brings ecstasy and rapture. Moreover, devotional mantras are available to everyone without too many rules and regulations about their usage. This accessibility made Bhava Yoga the devotional elixir of the masses.

VAISHNAVISM AND THE DEVOTIONAL PATH OF BHAKTI

The term "Bhava Yoga" is best associated with the *Vaishnava* tradition, an orthodox branch of Hinduism that goes back to the inception of the Vedic age. Although some of their cultural beliefs were questionable, such as their strong sense of caste and the requirement that widows self-immolate upon the death of their husbands, the Vaishnavas built their tradition on an intense love relationship between the human soul and the Divine; theirs is a path of ecstatic love and rapturous union. Vaishnavism develops around

Vishnu, the one who pervades and preserves the universe. In Vaishnavism, we find all the principles of sacred sound that we've studied; Vak, the parts of the syllable Om signifying states of consciousness, and the various stages of linguistic expression are all found in mystical relationship to Vishnu. While Shabda Brahman is perceived to be the ultimate principle of the universe, the alphabet and vowels are associated with Lakshmi, Vishnu's shakti and feminine counterpart. For Vaishnavas, Lakshmi is the "mother of all sound."[1] Vishnu and Lakshmi form the hearth of the householder's devotion because, together, these deities preserve the well-being of the household and generate abundance and wealth for the family and the community.

In the Bhakti cults of devotional yoga, Vishnu, incarnating through the beauty of Krishna and the righteous reign of Rama, allows the Divine to become human. Of course, Shiva and Shakti have their devotees, too. What is special about Vaishnava Bhakti is the intensity of the devotion. Attributes associated with Vishnu, Krishna, Rama, and Sita became a powerful means of infusing the same attributes into the soul of the devotee. Many of these universal Divine attributes can also be found in mantras associated with Shiva, Ganesha, or the Great Goddess Shakti. All Hindus, whether worshippers of Vishnu, Shiva, or Shakti, believe that ultimately there is only one Supreme Being who transcends both name and form; devotion to a specific name or form is based only on circumstantial need and the personality of the yogi or devotee.

The power of the Bhakti tradition was that it offered the ordinary householder a means of liberation from suffering and the endless cycle of birth and death. This liberation is essentially gained through chanting and singing the holy names of personal deities, praising their attributes to infuse them into the soul of the devotee, and celebrating the deities' interventions in human suffering. This devotional stream of sacred sound continues to be prevalent throughout India as the grassroots spirituality of the working classes. While mantra shastra, the science of mantra, is also prevalent in the Vaishnava tradition, its complex rules and rituals are practiced only by the Brahmin, or priestly, community, as mentioned before. *Kirtana,* a common and widespread practice of Sound Yoga that originated in the Bhakti tradition, has in recent years become extremely popular in yoga studios across America in the form of the call-and-response chanting called *kirtan*.

Kirtan and Kirtana

"KIRTANA," which means "chanting the holy names of God and singing songs about God," was the means through which the Bhakti movement spread throughout India during the Middle Ages. Many of the spiritual catalysts of this movement — musician saints and poets such as Kabir, Mirabai, and Tukaram — are now well-known in the West. One point of confusion is that kirtans are not always composed of mantras. In the Hindu system, only certain words and sounds qualify as mantras, although many words and phrases may "function" as mantras. There is obviously a difference. Certain kirtans and spiritual songs, for instance, may refer to Divine exploits mentioned in mythological stories. Such phrases would not be considered to have the same power as mantras that directly embody the essence or attributes of a deity; the exploits only tell about the deity. Yet, if repeated over and over, such kirtans would have a mantra-like effect.

It is also important to realize that many kirtans and spiritual songs were written in regional languages — Bengali, Gujarati, Marati, Hindi — that are derived from Sanskrit. Because Sanskrit was known only by the priestly and administrative castes, this is how the Bhakti movement spread throughout the country and became accessible to everyone, including the illiterate villager. Like modern English, the sounds of these vernacular tongues, although derived from the original mantric power of the Sanskrit language, became adulterated through colloquialisms and adaptations. Even the classical Sanskrit of literature would be considered less mantric in its power than the old Vedic Sanskrit. From the mantric point of view, one may describe the comparisons using sugar as a metaphor. Ancient Vedic Sanskrit is like raw sugar; classical Sanskrit is like refined white sugar; and the vernacular derivatives are like synthetic sugar substitutes. Tantric bijas, on the other hand, are like molasses; they are the purest, most intense form of mantra.

But even in light of this important comparison — one that few propagators of mantras in the West are truly knowledgeable about — kirtans and Hindu spiritual songs in regional languages have a unique spiritual power. The yearning for union, for yoga, described in these beautiful lyrical passages, and the haunting melodies that go with them, effortlessly transport the yogi into a profound state of union with the Deity. Once in that mystic union, why argue about whether the lyrical sounds used to get there were mantras or not?

A famous story from the life of Shankaracharya, one of Hinduism's greatest philosophers who lived in the eighth century A.D., sets the record straight about the power of devotion — a power that I trust and believe in from my own experience. Coming upon a brahmin priest struggling to master the rules of grammar, Shankara cries out: "Sing with devotion the name of God, you fool! Of what use will your rules of grammar be at the appointed hour of death?"

The point to remember, though, is that Vedic and Tantric mantras do have rules, and pronunciation is indeed important with these types of mantras. Westerners tend to confuse Vedic and Tantric mantras with kirtana, and this corrupts the power of their sound and function. The hundreds — perhaps thousands — of years of research that have gone into sculpting these amazing sounds are disregarded and lost in the sometimes frivolous adaptation to contemporary tunes and the domestication of the primal power of these mantras.

I am not a purist. I do believe in the evolution of art and spirituality. But I also believe that the process should not sacrifice power, depth, and function, as you will discover in any of my yoga music albums. My hope, in bringing out the full scope of the Yoga of Sound in this literary work, is that it will encourage Western yogis to gradually develop mantric power through their systematic effort. If Western yogis employ even one-tenth of the effort that they put into their asana practice in the proper application and pronunciation of Vedic and Tantric mantras, they will gain a tremendous depth of realization.

SINGING FOR GOD

THE MESMERIZING melodies and mystical power of kirtans and Hindu devotional songs are derived from sacred Hindu *ragas.* Ragas are specific sequences of musical intervals with distinctive musical nuances that evoke particular shades of spiritual emotion. Each raga serves to enhance, deepen, and nurture the soul's relationship with the Divine through its unique tonal characteristics. The soul's longing for union with the Divine, the bliss of that union when it happens, the pain of separation — all of these conditions are exquisitely portrayed and lived to the fullest through the song and chant expressed in the raga.

While musical knowledge is helpful for drawing out the subtleties of human emotions, many practitioners of devotional yoga are able to penetrate to the heart of this union, even with a crackly voice and no ability to carry a tune. It is their intense desire and yearning for the Beloved that breaks through all barriers.

The greatest asset a sound yogi has is his or her voice, which has been provided as a tool for self-realization, empowerment, and the expression of joy. Through song, we open and lift up our heart to the Divine. I often meet people who, in childhood, were told not to sing because their voice wasn't good enough or because they were considered tone-deaf. Bhava Yoga is a powerful way to heal the wounded singer who dwells in many of us; the singer is the healer, as in the Shamanic traditions. Bhava Yoga is not about performance; it is not about impressing an audience, or for that matter even impressing ourselves. It is about singing for God and pouring out the deepest sentiments of our soul into a conscious awareness of the Divine presence.

A classic story exemplifying the spirit of Bhava Yoga comes to us from the thirteenth century. Tan Sen was the chief court musician of the great Mogul emperor Akbar, a passionate patron of the arts with a keen interest in world spirituality. Tan Sen was an expert in Hindustani music, the Persian-influenced form of Indian music that developed in Northern India where the Mughals ruled.

Curious about where Tan Sen disappeared to on certain days of the month, the Emperor made inquiries and discovered that he went to be with his music teacher. Akbar, who never let an opportunity to hear great music pass him by, asked Tan Sen to arrange for his master to perform at court. "I'm sorry, your majesty," was Tan Sen's reply. "My teacher is a yogi who lives in a remote cave. His lifestyle and spiritual practice keep him absorbed in the woods. He rarely ventures outside the forest."

Akbar, now desperate, wanted to go to this yogi. But Tan Sen refused to take the king, explaining that his majesty's retinue of servants and horses would only drive the yogi deeper into the forest, perhaps never to be found again. Finally it was agreed that the king would disguise himself as Tan Sen's solitary servant and carry a musical instrument on the journey.

As they neared the cave, Akbar stopped in his tracks and inhaled deeply. A pleasant feeling came over him; he looked almost intoxicated. Slowly, the king began to turn. Round and round he turned, throwing up his arms and rolling his head in ecstasy until he fell down exhausted. Hours later, Akbar awoke from his deep sleep and looked around. Everything seemed to have changed. The leaves looked brighter, the sounds of the birds were more melodious, and there was lightness in his heart.

"Oh, Tan Sen," he exclaimed, "all I could hear was a raspy voice singing a raga that I've heard you sing many times in court. But never have I felt this way! Why is this so?"

"Your majesty," replied Tan Sen, "while you have commissioned me to sing exclusively at your court, my master has commissioned himself to sing exclusively at God's."

BHAVA YOGA AND MUSIC

Bhava Yoga relies on the rich, dynamic use of music. Indian classical music, one of the oldest and most sophisticated musical traditions in the world, originated between the fifth and ninth centuries A.D., escalated in development in the Middle Ages through its interaction with the Persian musical strains brought into the country by Muslims. Bhava yogis, called *bhaktas* because of their intense devotion to a particular God or Goddess, used not only the sophisticated classical music traditions — the ancient indigenous Carnatic music of the South as well as the Persian-influenced Hindustani of the North — but also the simple folk melodies of the rice fields and the mountains. Such melodies had been in use for many hundreds of years and were the roots of Indian classical music, in the same way that gospel and blues are the basis for modern jazz and pop in the West.

Indian classical music itself can be considered a sophisticated expression of Bhava Yoga, with its spiritual principles founded on Nada Yoga, the stream we will explore in the next chapter. Yet one need not be a musical expert to enjoy the experience of Bhava, which is a quality of the heart. In fact, too much technical knowledge of music could become an obstacle to the interior journey.

The musicality of Bhava Yoga sets it in stark contrast to the three other streams. You will recall that the Vedic mantras of Shabda Yoga are typically chanted with just three musical intervals, one higher and one lower than the base tone. Shakti Yoga mantras, on the other hand, are generally not sung unless they are being expressed devotionally. Bija mantras, for example, are never sung.

Music is a powerful means of opening the heart, often piercing it to the core. The most popular form of devotional chanting, kirtan, employs an ingenious yoga technique in which the leader sings a phrase and the group repeats it; a variation is sung, and the group echoes the variation. The variations, which could be either predictable or unpredictable, allows for constant change in the style, meter, rhythm, melody, and even lyrics. It is a wonderful form of meditation, because it keeps both the chant leader and those responding fully alert in the moment, while at the same time sustaining an uninterrupted flow of energy between the chanters and the Divine. This devotional connection can be maintained for a prolonged period, even by poor meditators.

In chapter one, we discussed the imbalance caused by modern culture, which coerces us to live and function solely from the left, analytical brain. We also learned that yoga, according to Patanjali's *Yoga Sutras,* is the cessation of the modifications of the mind — notably linear, discursive thinking. Devotional chant and kirtan provide a simple method of sustaining right-brain activity for an extended period. Quite simply, variations in melody and rhythm stimulate the feminine brain of the practitioner. In India, this sort of devotional chanting often goes on all night.

BHAVA AND RITUAL

Evenings are the best time for devotional yoga practice. After a long day's work, we want comfort and relationship; we want to express our pain or frustration at events that didn't go well, and give thanks for those that did. Bhava Yoga allows us to surrender the fruits of our labor as a selfless offering to the Beloved, and to seek the Divine embrace, often through ritual. We have largely lost our capacity for personal ritual in the West, conferring most of its power upon priests. In Hinduism, the technology of ritual is an essential way of caring for the soul. When performed regularly, ritual can release the accumulation of psychic toxicity in our spiritual system.

Ritual, although not imperative in any of the streams of sacred sound, is the backbone of the Yoga of Sound tradition. For eons, it has provided the human family with a medium that accommodates the full spectrum of human and spiritual emotion in a safe container. Although we have all but banished it from Western culture, ritual is what holds a community together, heals it, and allows it to transform into a spiritual entity. Ritual is about expressing grief and joy; it is about going both deep and high; it is about facing our communal shadow and embracing our communal soul. We need personal as well as communal rituals to enhance our spiritual lives, and Bhava Yoga offers us a way to do this.

A Bhava Yoga Ritual

1. Take a quick shower to purify your body. Dress in comfortable white clothes — a color used to represent inner purity. Gather about ten to twenty small flowers, or remove the petals of a larger flower to obtain this number. You can also use a bunch of leaves or blades of grass. Put these in a basket or arrange them on a plate; they will be used to express your devotion. Keep a small pitcher of water — preferably one that has a spout — near your meditation seat.
2. For your altar, place your personal deity in front of you; it could be a statue of Krishna, a photograph of the Buddha, a crucifix, even a special stone or sacred object that is particularly meaningful to you. You may also use a photograph of

someone dear to you, such as a lover, a teacher, a child, or a parent. If you prefer not to use an image, you can sit before an open window overlooking a garden, a body of water, or the open sky.

3. Pour a small quantity of water into the palm of your right hand and sip it. Visualize your mind being purified. Sprinkle some water around the place where you are sitting and visualize your meditation seat being cleared of any undesirable emotions. Finally, sprinkle some water around your altar and visualize a wall of fire springing up around your place of worship; this fire will protect you from all negative energy throughout the ceremony.

4. Take a flower, petal, or leaf in your right hand and place it on your heart. If your personal deity is masculine, say, "Lord, I love you" and place the flower at the foot of his image; you may also place the flower between you and the image, or directly upon it. If the image is feminine, you may say, "Mother, I adore you," or "Goddess, I worship you." If it is a child, you could say, "My child, I embrace you with all my heart." These phrases are just examples of how you can express your devotion; you can always express this devotion to life itself or to the unseen presence of the Divine, without shape or form. The objective is to stimulate love and devotion in your heart, and to do so meaningfully. See the beginning of appendix three for a devotional mantra litany that can be used with this ritual.

5. Since you will be doing this practice in private, I encourage you to sing as you place the flower or leaf on your heart and then on the image. St. Augustine once wrote that "those who sing pray twice." Tones evoke emotion. Don't be overly concerned about whether you can sing or whether you have a pleasing voice. Remember the tuneless song that wins a heart in romance, or the crackly voice of a mother soothing her baby to sleep? The soul does not judge, nor does it compare. Spirit doesn't either. Only the personality

does that. When you sing, you evoke your soul. Don't let your personality keep you from doing that. A couple of tonal sequences are also featured for the mantra litany in appendix three.

6. Get into the experience and keep it simple. Maintain eye contact with the image or keep your eyes closed; you can even alternate between closed and open eyes in a way that feels natural.
7. Follow step four with each flower, one by one, slowly and mindfully conscious of every action and of the energy being built up by your devotion. At times, words may not come to your mind. That's okay; just place the flower silently and lovingly in front of you. The petals or leaves could also be arranged in a pattern or cast lovingly upon the image. Don't get too caught up in what might be correct; be natural, spontaneous, present, open, and soft.
8. When you feel satiated with love and devotion, sit quietly and allow the energy you are experiencing to infuse every layer of your being.

Manasika Puja

If you can't put together the ingredients for the ritual, you can always create the entire experience in your mind, using your imagination. Then you can offer gold, precious stones, beautifully crafted ornaments, and generous quantities of grain. *Manasika Puja* means "mental ritual." Traditionally, because Vishnu helps us find support in our worldly lives, he is offered sweets and rich, buttery offerings. On the other hand, Shiva, the God of yogis, is offered fruits and shoots. The fierce aspect of Shakti, the goddess, is offered lemon and chilies, while her healing presence is offered turmeric.

If you open up your heart
You will know what I mean
We've been polluted so long
But here's a way for you to get clean

By chanting the names of the Lord and you'll be free
The Lord is awaiting on you all to awaken and see.

— **George Harrison,**
"Awaiting On You All," from the album *All Things Must Pass*

BHAVA MANTRAS FOR WALKING AND JOGGING

ONE PART of the Vaishnava tradition that many Westerners have encountered is the Hare Krishna sect, which traces its lineage to Lord Chaitanya in the second century B.C. I have always been struck by their passionate love for the Divine, which they uninhibitedly express on the streets as they dance and chant in praise of Krishna. This uninhibited abandonment to the love of God is at the heart of Bhava Yoga and the Bhakti tradition. While we may not feel comfortable dressing in formal spiritual attire, wearing markings on our forehead, or dancing ecstatically in public, we can always chant mentally or whisper while we walk, run, or exercise. An excellent mantra to use while walking or jogging is the *Vaishnava Maha Mantra,* which means "great mantra." This rhythmic series of syllables — the same ones you may have heard the Hare Krishna devotees chanting — can serve to awaken tremendous joy and devotion in your heart in the midst of any activity:

Ha-re Raa-ma, Ha-re Raa-ma
Raa-ma, Raa-ma, Ha-re, Ha-re
Ha-re Krish-na, Ha-re Krish-na
Krish-na Krish-na, Ha-re, Ha-re

Rama and Krishna are both manifestations of Vishnu. According to the mystical interpretation of these mantric sounds, *Ram* is perceived to awaken joy in the heart, and *Krish* attracts because it embodies the power of the Divine to draw us unto itself.

You might remember that, in 1969, George Harrison recorded the Hare Krishna mantra with the devotees of the London Radha-Krishna Temple. Soon after rising to the top twenty on the best-selling record charts throughout England, Europe, and parts of Asia, the Hare Krishna chant became a familiar sound, especially in England.[2]

Another good walking and jogging mantra is:

Shree Raam, Jai Raam, Jai Jai Raamo

Shree is a title of respect, *Jai* is praise, and *Ram* is that which awakens joy in the heart. When writing this chapter, I contacted Mahatma Gandhi's grandson, Arun Gandhi, to determine the complete form of the Ram mantra that the Mahatma used. He graciously replied with the following devotional song in Hindi, which everyone sang at morning and evening prayer at Gandhi's ashram. This is a good example of a popular devotional chant, kirtana, which is not a mantra but can have a powerful effect upon our consciousness. Two versions of the song are available on my album, *Bhava Yoga*.

Ra-gu-pa-ṯi Raa-gha-va Raa-jaa Raam
Pa-ṯee-ṯa paa-va-na See-ṯaa Raam
See-ṯaa Raam jai See-ṯaa Raam
Ba-ja pyaa-re ṯo See-ṯaa Raam
Eesh-vara Allah ṯay-ro naam
Sabiko San-maṯi de Bha-ga-vaan

The shortened form of this chant is simply *Jai Ram,* or "praise Ram." Translated into English, the full version means:

Great king Ram of the Raghu clan,
Holy husband of Sita, the earth's daughter
We praise you joined in holiness as Sita Ram.
Let us sing together of your love,
Lord Ishvar, Allah, whichever name we call you,
It is still the same reality that we are addressing.

CHAPTER 10

NADA YOGA:
MEDITATION THROUGH SOUND AND MUSIC

At the root of all power and motion, there is music and rhythm, the play of patterned frequencies against the matrix of time. Before we make music, music makes us.

— ***George Leonard***[1]

"Nada Yoga" is the classical term for the Yoga of Sound in the Hindu tradition. It is a stream of sacred sound that embraces Hatha Yoga, the occult linguistics of Tantra, and the spirituality of classical Indian music. By including the nonlinguistic element of music, Nada Brahman augments the Shabda Brahman of the Vedic tradition, as well as the differentiation of energy in the chakras discovered by the Tantrics. While Bhava Yoga chooses only those frequencies that we classify as music in our earthly appreciation of sound, Nada yogis incorporate the full spectrum of frequencies — both those that are audible to the human ear and those that are inaudible — within the field of their yoga practice. This means that all forms of earthly music, the sounds of space, and even the entire electromagnetic spectrum of frequencies are included within this range of perception.

Human hearing lies in the range of between sixteen and twenty thousand hertz. "Frequency" refers to the number of wave cycles that occur in one second, giving rise to the experience of high and low tones. Wavelength gets longer as the frequency (or pitch) decreases. Although we may not "hear" all the frequencies that exist in our universe, we are affected by these waves at every moment, and we in turn affect these frequencies by our own sounds and activities.

What are the sounds of space? Throughout space, we find sounds emitted by such phenomena as the hum of planets, the gaseous states of the sun, and pulsating rhythms from the stars. Often, these sounds are similar to our earthly music. Phil Uttley and Ian McHardy of the University of Southampton, who have been studying the music of black holes in space, state: "If you were to transcribe the X-ray output of these black holes as a series of musical notes, it would not sound quite like any [particular] sort of music... but the 'tune' [would] still have a musical quality about it. The general pattern of note changes — the relative size of the changes in pitch from one note to the next, or from one bar to the next — are the same as one hears in all kinds of music." Uttley also claims that the music of a black hole could be called improvisational. The study further revealed that, at any given moment, various black holes are playing different styles of music — and every few weeks, a stellar black hole switches musical styles, undergoing a distinct transition from one pattern of variability to another.[2]

As mentioned earlier, the tradition of Nada Yoga does not specialize in the mantra shastras of the other streams. For instance, it doesn't deal with rituals governing mantras or their pronunciation, mystical meanings, or embodiment of energy. However, Nada Yoga does bring together all the key elements and cosmogonies of sacred sound that are explored in those streams, including the devotional element of Bhava, represented in Nada Yoga by the tradition of Indian classical music. In the first millennium B.C., Nada yogis focused extensively on the mantra *Om,* which Patanjali's classic *Yoga Sutras* teach is the "sound that expresses the Divine Absolute," which should be "repeatedly intoned while absorbing its meaning."[3] In chapter fourteen, we will explore this unitive capacity of the sacred syllable *Om,* which summarizes all mantric knowledge. Since the Middle Ages, Nada yogis proficient in music have combined India's rapidly evolving musical system with the sonic cosmology and philosophy of Tantra and the Vedas. But it is only in the past few centuries that the strongest connections between music and Nada Yoga have been established.

Interestingly, despite the fact that "Nada Yoga" is the classical term for the Yoga of Sound, and despite many contemporary Indian musicians using the term "Nada Yoga" to describe the profound spiritual significance of their musical disciplines, Nada Yoga as a well-defined practice is perhaps the least documented of all the streams of sacred sound. There are references to Nada Yoga practices in a number of scriptures, which I will soon address, but the approach is not as organized or synthesized as that of Hatha Yoga. Many musicians and yogis in the West casually refer to sacred sound in yoga as "Nada Yoga" without realizing that the term does not deal effectively with the phonetic subtleties of mantra. It is precisely for this reason that I prefer to use the term "Yoga of Sound" to refer to the full scope of sacred sound and its evolution in yoga. What is specific to Nada Yoga, and where we will find its unique benefits, is its understanding of the process of meditation using sound as its essential medium.

SOUND AS FLOWING CURRENT

As a tradition, Nada Yoga originates with the codification of the *Yoga Sutras* of Patanjali in the second century and closely parallels the development of Hatha Yoga. References to the use of sound in Hatha Yoga and Raja Yoga practice are found in texts such as the *Nada-Bindu Upanishad,* attached to the *Rg Veda,* and the *Hatha Yoga Pradipika,** a compendium of mystical writings held particularly sacred by Hatha yogis. These references essentially involve the use of the mantra *Om* in conjunction with focused listening techniques and audible breathing practices, which we will explore.

The word "nada" means "a loud sounding or droning or rushing," and it can refer to any sound, whether linguistic or nonlinguistic.

* The *Nada-Bindu Upanishad* is perhaps the oldest document on sacred sound, dating from between 500 and 200 B.C. The *Hatha Yoga Pradipika* was authored by the great sage Svatmarama in 1400 A.D.

Although Nada Yoga does not deal with the particularities of mantra shastra present in other streams of sacred sound, it is like the underlying current present in all those streams, carrying them toward the great ocean of consciousness. Musicologist Joachim-Ernst Berendt points out that the names of many rivers around the world are based on the word "nada." The Norwegian Nid, the German Nidda, and the Polish Nida are just a few examples. Because of its etymological associations, "nada" is best translated as "currents of sound" that exist in the human body and in the universe. Nada Yoga offers an internal experience of sound frequencies by means of meditation, induced by the external sound of vocal and instrumental music. In other words, when entertainment leads to "innertainment," music becomes yoga.

Nada Yoga's feminine qualities — being a fluid, interior, sensual practice — complement the more rigid Shabda Yoga. Attunement is a primary aspect of Nada Yoga; the flowing currents in our body — especially our emotions — can be adjusted to the frequencies and tones used by the practitioner. This is why the ascent and descent of the voice or musical instrument on a musical scale — DO, RE, MI, FA, SO, LA, TI, DO — is a Nada Yoga practice. Ascending the musical scale (ascending in pitch) harmonically configures our emotions and channels them toward Divine union, which is considered to be a higher and more rapid vibratory frequency.

There is yet to be a thorough study of Nada Yoga, but great credit should be given to musicologist Guy L. Beck, who has collected an excellent summary of esoteric texts in his seminal work *Sonic Theology*,[4] which I reference in this and other chapters.

THE SCIENCE OF SOUND

The cosmology of Nada Yoga embraces the notion that the primary stuff of the universe is vibratory, and therefore sonic in nature. Modern physics supports this understanding, especially via the new field of string theory, which claims that the entire universe may be made up of infinitesimally small subatomic strands of energy vibrating at different frequencies. These cosmologies all recognize that the shapes we see in nature are constructed of vibrating entities, each with a different frequency and wavelength. The speed at which an object vibrates (as well as its size, however infinitesimal) contributes to its particular sound. I mentioned earlier that solid objects vibrate relatively slowly, while gaseous substances vibrate more rapidly. Thus, the tones and frequencies that comprise the known universe become the subject of meditation in Nada Yoga. This science of Nada Yoga, which also takes into consideration the musical intervals used in music and in the musical recitation of mantras, is brought together with meditation techniques and certain Hatha Yoga practices that are conducive to sonic exploration.

Nada Yoga involves a deep listening to the body, to its inner sounds and acoustics. Nada Yoga also includes listening deeply to the music of the natural world. We can perceive a lot of sound-based creative activity in nature, such as the mating calls of birds and the amazingly complex and sonorous whale song. Such listening reveals the vast spectrum of consciousness, which manifests in a wide range of distinct frequencies during meditation. Our musical systems across the globe — the varied senses of harmony, melody, and rhythm — are all selections from this vast range of frequencies. But to choose only a portion of these frequencies narrows us to restricted cultural boundaries. Jean Houston explains, "Every person has a different tonality and is made up of different sonar frequencies. That is why we prefer different things and are so radically different from and to each other. We must not impose, as let's say a Wagnerian derived music, a limitation of mind through a sonar imprisonment of people. This politicizing of brain function through various kinds of sounds and forms is not only what happened in Germany, but also occurs whenever and wherever totalitarian states and dictators prevail."[5]

The practice of Nada Yoga can help broaden the consciousness of an audience. For instance, the Western ear, trained and conditioned by tempered intervals, came to perceive other music as inferior or out of tune; only in recent years, with the rapid surge of world music, have ethnic sounds, non-Western musical intervals, variable instrument tunings, and diverse musical scales "enlarged" the Western ear. The power of cultivating a larger ear has never been more necessary than it is now; it will result in a proportionately larger heart, facilitating an authentic acceptance of other cultures and their vibrations.

THE UNSTRUCK SOUND

MANY TREATISES on the practice of Nada Yoga describe various stages of listening to the body via the right ear. For instance, the *Nada-Bindu Upanishad* describes a process of yogic meditation in which the aspirant listens to eleven different internal sounds with successive degrees of subtlety:

> *The yogis should always listen to the sound [nada] in the interior of the right ear. This sound, when constantly practiced, will drown every external sound [dhvani] from the outside. . . . By persisting . . . the sound will be heard subtler and subtler. At first, it will be like what is produced by the ocean, the cloud, the kettledrum, and the waterfall. . . . A little later it will be like the sound produced by a small drum, a big bell, and a military drum; and finally like the sound of a tinkling bell, the bamboo flute, the harp, and the bee.*[6]

The point of the exercise is to keep the yogi listening, because as we get closer to the inner experience of sound in our body, the sound starts to change. Another scripture, the *Darsana Upanishad,* describes the perception of sounds in the highest position or chakra in the body, referred to here as the Brahma-randa, located at the crown of the head.

> *When air [prana] enters the Brahma-randa, nada [sound] is also produced there, resembling at first the sound of a conch-blast and then like the thunder-clap in the middle; and when the air has reached the middle of the head, like the roaring of a mountain cataract. Thereafter, O great wise one! The Atman [indwelling Divine Presence], mightily pleased, will actually appear in front of thee. Then there will be the ripeness of the knowledge of the Spirit from yoga and the disowning by the yogi of worldly existence.*[7]

While many of these passages seem esoteric, or even fanciful on occasion, they all point to a sonic universe that reveals itself to us as we become increasingly attuned to it. About twenty years ago, I read *The Prophet,*[8] by Lebanese mystic Kahlil Gibran; you are no doubt familiar with this extraordinary mystical treatise. I was just beginning to explore the Yoga of Sound at that time, and I was profoundly struck by this statement: "A seeker of silences am I, and what treasure have I found in silences that I may dispense with confidence?" Earlier, he also wrote, "Then the gates of his heart were flung open, and his joy flew far over the sea. And he closed his eyes and prayed in the silences of his soul." Notice, Gibran does not say *silence,* which is typical of such writings, but he uses the plural, *silences.* The difference helps us understand Nada Yoga meditation.

Silence, generally speaking, is the absence of noise. For most of us, living a busy life in the world, "noise" refers to external sounds that we're not in control of: traffic, generators, the humming of appliances. We take a trip into the countryside to gain some peace and quiet, away from these sounds, where we discover that a remarkable quiet pervades nature. What precisely enables the ear to hear sounds? Physically and biologically, the process is described in terms of sound waves, produced by various oscillating structures, traveling through the medium of air. The ear receives these waves, processes them, and sends them on as impulses to the brain. Just as the ear recognizes individual sounds that register in its field of perception, we also know that it can recognize silence. What is silence? Does it have its own sound?

Mystics of the ancient world perceived all individual sounds as taking place against a background of unheard silence behind the sounds. In Nada Yoga, this background is called *anahata* nada, meaning the "unstruck sound." Anahata is the name for the heart chakra in Kundalini or Shakti Yoga. As Nada yogis, we are therefore urged to listen with the "ear of the heart," a phrase also used in the Benedictine way of monastic life.

What, then, is unstruck sound? The friction of objects generally causes explicit sounds, but the constant backdrop of silence is not a struck sound; it is the "sound of space." Space is the unseen medium in which we experience the movement of all energy. And silence — the sound of this space — is as vast, pervasive, and indestructible as the space itself. Sounds and vibrations magically arise from and disappear back into it. Quantum physicists call it the field of indeterminate particles, because we cannot predict exactly where particles will show up next. Sufis refer to this silent space as *Zat,* meaning "the silent life" from which all vibrations arise and into which all vibrations dissolve; an exact parallel to the findings of quantum physicists. Buddhists call this space *sunnyata,* the void, and Hindus call it Nada Brahman, the soundless sound that *is* God. When compared to the Shabda Brahman of the Vedas, we can say that Shabda Brahman is the eternal Word that issues forth from the Divine mouth, and Nada Brahman is the eternal music that is sounding in the Divine heart.

Hindu mystics, especially Nada yogis, identify many levels of silence. The first level is the immediate backdrop that makes it possible to hear the sounds we hear. As we begin to listen to this silence, we realize that we can "hear" it only because another backdrop exists behind it. In exploring these unfolding layers of silence, we become, like Gibran, seekers of silences, with each level registering its own unique vibratory signal. Thus we may hear frequencies analogous to kettledrums and ocean waves, thunder and waterfalls.

THE SOUND OF SILENCE

ONE PRACTICE of interior silences that we shall explore in Nada Yoga is called *Brahmari mudra.* The term *brahmari* derives from the bee-like buzzing sound produced by the yogi during this practiçe, which is performed using a six-way seal of body apertures known as *shanmukhi mudra* or *yoni mudra.* This sealing of apertures involves filtering sound by pressing the thumbs against both ear canals, preventing light from entering the two eyes using the index and middle fingers, and blocking air from entering the nostrils using the two ring fingers. Please see appendix four for a detailed description of this practice.

Using sound in yoga practice often means noticing what sound reveals. Mantras and music both reveal something, and this something arises in the stillness and silence that follow the sound. The quiet at the end of a symphony is a good example of the yogic poise produced by the various musical movements. A symphony is like a yoga routine; the essence of the experience is absorbed by the soul at the end of whole performance. Even in Vedic mantras, you will recall that the Veda (shabda) is both sruti and smriti — that which is heard and that which is revealed.

The *Shiva Samhita,* an ancient yogic treatise, describes a type of brahmari as follows:

> *Let him [the yogi or yogini] close the ears with his thumbs... this is my most beloved yoga. From practicing this gradually, the yogi begins to hear mystic sounds [nadas]. The first is like the hum of the honey-intoxicated bee, next that of a flute, then of a harp; after this, by the gradual practice of yoga, the destroyer of the darkness of the world, he hears the sound of ringing bells; then sounds like the roar of thunder. When one fixes his full attention on this sound, being free from fear, the yogi gets absorption [in Divine Bliss].*[9]

The *Hatha Yoga-Pradipika* declares that the worship of Nada Brahman is an essential practice for Hatha yogis. The text proclaims that the hearing of anahata nada (unstruck sound) is paramount among the millions of trance-inducing practices propounded by Shiva himself:

> *The Yogi should hear the sound inside his right ear, with collected mind. The ears, the eyes, the nose, and the mouth should be closed, and then the clear sound is heard in the passage of the susumna [central channel], which has been cleansed of all its impurities.*[10]

HARMONY: MUSIC AS MEDICINE

All music, in one way or another, is therapeutic because it can heal. Behind this healing are the principles of Nada Yoga: the notion that sound is God — that sound is holy, and therefore capable of restoring wholeness. Around the world, from Greece to Egypt to India, cultures have used music to restore health and harmony in a system out of balance. We mentioned earlier the temple of Asclepius, to which Hippocrates took his patients to give them music as a form of therapy. Music therapists who continue this noble work have had remarkable results in their healing ministry. The music most used by Western therapists is harmonic music with rhythmic patterns. My hope is that melody and mantra will be included in future medical research and healing. When we understand the three musical aspects of harmony, rhythm, and melody, we can grasp the essential teaching of Nada Yoga, which we can then apply toward our own healing and that of others. The following explanation will help a nonmusician understand how this works.

When we hear a certain frequency — a note played on an instrument, the hum of a generator, or the prolonged tone of a singer — the wavelength of that particular sound moving through the medium of air affects our bodies, causing our cells and tissues to vibrate in unison with the tone of the vibrating body. In other words, our body resonates with that particular tone, which is known as the "fundamental tone" or, interestingly, "the tonic." The tonic can be any frequency. When another tone, different from the fundamental tone, is simultaneously generated, a certain tension is established. This is called a "musical interval." Human beings experience some of these intervals as pleasant and enjoyable; we call these "consonant intervals." Those that feel uncomfortable and jarring we call "dissonant."

When you begin with a given frequency and keep increasing it (raising its pitch), the original frequency will eventually double. This new pitch will sound similar to the fundamental tone even though it is vibrating at a different rate. We call the distance between these two frequencies the "octave." Between these two frequencies that make up the octave, we have identified eleven other frequencies at specific distances from each other, giving us a total of twelve distances or intervals. These are the tempered intervals — equal divisions of the octave — I mentioned earlier, which are used in popular music in the West. Seven of these combinations (the fundamental plus one of the eleven frequencies) are considered consonant, while five are considered dissonant. Some are more consonant or dissonant than others.

The following chart illustrates how and why these tones range from increased consonance to increased dissonance. You will notice that the ratios (which represent the frequencies in relation to the fundamental) are gradually moving away from wholeness. The human ear seems to prefer whole numbers, and this conveys the experience of increased consonance or dissonance to the rest of the body. Simpler ratios are more harmonious. The broken line divides the upper (consonant) intervals from the lower (dissonant) intervals; the names for these intervals in Western music theory is given beside each ratio:

CONSONANCE-TO-DISSONANCE SEQUENCE

1:1 unison

1:2 octave

2:3	fifth
3:4	fourth
3:5	major sixth
4:5	major third
5:6	minor third
5:8	minor sixth
5:9	minor seventh
8:9	major second
8:15	major seventh
15:16	minor second
32:45	augmented fourth or tritone

The ratios listed above are critical to understanding harmony as it exists at every level of being in our universe. Joachim-Ernst Berendt points out that consonant sounds — proportions made up mainly of low whole numbers — are highly prevalent in our universe, at macroscopic as well as at microscopic levels. What is truly astonishing is the fact that our world is not only made up of sounds, but that these sounds are overwhelmingly harmonious. Berendt writes:

> *Not only the planetary orbits, but also the proportions within these orbits follow the laws of harmonics, much more so than statistical probability would lead us to expect . . . out of the seventy-eight tones created by the different planetary proportions, seventy-four belong to the major scale."*[11]

This major scale is the most consonant series of musical intervals that we know and use in our music. According to Berendt, the most frequent consonance is also the most harmonious, namely the octave. This proportion, 1:2, has always been used to signify the polarity and balance of the world: yang and yin, male and female, heaven and earth.* Furthermore, this yogic ratio is not only "written into the sky," but also in our ears, because our ears prefer consonance (major proportions) to dissonance.[12]

* One part — the Divine, completes two parts — the perfectly equal or balanced male and female combination. Thus, 1:2 is the most consonant of ratios.

Now, if you were to move step by step from the fundamental tone toward the octave, the intervals just listed would occur in the order shown in the following chart. This is their natural sequence, and it is exactly the order in which they occur on properly tuned piano keys or guitar frets. Each step is called a half-step or half-tone; two of these intervals spaced side by side make up a whole step or whole tone.

THE CHROMATIC SEQUENCE

Base tone (the fundamental) resonates in unison	**1:1**
minor second	15:16
major second	8:9
minor third	5:6
major third	4:5
fourth	3:4
tritone	32:45 (aka augmented fourth)
fifth	**2:3**
minor sixth	5:8
major sixth	3:5
minor seventh	5:9
major seventh	8:15
octave	**1:2**

Notice that there is a minor and a major option for all intervals, except for the fundamental, the fifth, and the octave, which appear in boldface. These are called "perfect intervals." All the others have a sharped or flatted option, which means that interval can be raised or lowered in pitch by a half-step. Thus, DO, RE, MI, FA, SO, LA, TI, and DO are the eight intervals of the octave, but five of them — RE, MI, FA, LA, and TI — have the option of being sharped or flatted. By choosing specific intervals to play simultaneously, we get a chord, which could be harmonious or disharmonious depending on how we combine these intervals.

Jazz music, for instance, stretches our musical ear to include many combinations of consonant and dissonant intervals. This is why it is sometimes called "atonal" music. Musical harmony, which comes to us through Western classical music, is derived from an understanding of chords that are structured with consonant intervals. Bach, Debussy, and Beethoven combined musical intervals in many ingenious ways, helping the Western ear gradually perceive harmony, even in intervals previously perceived as dissonant. Only the minor second, major second, tritone, minor seventh, and major seventh remain dissonant to our ears today. Harmonic music is therefore based on the relationship of simultaneous notes.

Melody, on the other hand, is the relationship of successive notes. All ancient music is, first and foremost, melodic. Celtic music and Gregorian chant, which is based on the ancient Greek modes, reveal this process. Indian music was the only type of music that remained melodic and developed melodic music to a high degree of sophistication. When you move from one note to another on a musical instrument, or when you sing or hum a tune, you *feel* the relationship between the notes; this is melody.

Played successively, the intervals rearranged on the second list — the chromatic sequence — are all a half-step from one another, and not as tuneful as a true melody. On the other hand, when you select a sequence of intervals such as the fundamental, the major second, the major third, the fourth, the fifth, the major sixth, and the major seventh, you have a melodious sequence. This particular sequence is the major scale mentioned earlier — the most consonant series in popular Western music, known to the Greeks as the Ionian mode. It is also the sequence sung by Julie Andrews to teach the von Trapp family fundamentals of music in *The Sound of Music.* She uses the Western musical syllable for each interval in the form of puns to teach them the sequence: DO, RE, MI, FA, SO, LA, TI, DO. The final do is half the wavelength of the fundamental DO.

There are many modal sequences like this and, as mentioned earlier, you can choose other intervals for the syllables RE, MI, FA, LA, and TI instead of those in the major scale sequence; this will give you a different tune. These choices of intervals allow music to convey a variety of emotions, awakening us to joy, sadness, melancholy, discomfort, strength, or comfort, and allowing us to create appropriate music to accompany movies, songs, operas, and musicals. This is also how we heal our souls and our bodies with music.

A specific set of intervals between the fundamental and the octave — say five, six, or seven notes — is called a "scale" in contemporary popular music, or a "mode" in ancient Western music. In Indian music and in Nada Yoga, this sequence of intervals is called a "raga."

RAGA: THE DEITIC ASPECT OF MUSIC

Ragas are the basis of Nada Yoga's musical expression. Like mantras, they can be used as tools for healing and the transformation of consciousness. In a broad sense, musicians are logically Nada yogis. Even though they may not be aware of the cosmology and the profound spiritual principles underlying their work, they are either consciously or unconsciously striving for harmony. Harmony, we know, is the goal of the universe. Since the last century, however, I believe that art for art's sake has disrupted this natural tendency, leading to a new breed of artists and empowering them with unrestricted license to propagate excessive violence and hatred through their art forms. This needs to change. I believe that artists — like politicians, business executives, and spiritual leaders — need to become more accountable for their choices and expressions. The only way this can happen is for spirituality to inform art, and vice versa.

In the fall of 1999, I spent a week with his holiness the Dalai Lama and about 150 other leaders in the arts, sciences, media, religion, business, and educational sectors of world society. We gathered at the Norbulingka Institute, in the foothills of the Himalayas, to discuss the role of spirituality in all these areas and to forge a synthesized perspective of independent disciplines, using spirituality as our common theme. I asked His Holiness what advice he had for artists today. "Learn to deal with your inner issues in private," he said. "Don't burden society with them; it is burdened enough. Transform your own energy first, then use your gifts to bring healing to society."

Musicians and artists all have to become yogis. We need to use our art to transform, not to self-destruct. We need to find healthy ways of handling the intense energy we process through our systems. Because artists work toward developing a refined sensitivity, they are also very vulnerable. I believe that the study of ragas as a spiritual practice, along with the chanting of mantras, can help greatly in our transformation and empowerment.

Ragas are analogous to musical scales and modes, but they are much more than a mere assortment of notes. Ragas are special sets of musical intervals with explicit ascending and descending orders; they are also governed by precise rules, which emphasize specific intervals and note combinations within each series. The Indian octave is divided into twenty-two srutis, or tones, offering the musician and the listener a subtle tonal system. The South Indian system of Carnatic music classifies 34,776 discrete ragas through a formula known as *Katyapadi Sankhya,* as well as countless *misra* ragas — mixed ragas that borrow notes within this well-defined system. What is more, ragas are worshipped as spiritual presences with distinctive personalities that come alive. Ancient Hindu sages declared: "Ragas are a coloring of the spirit."

All music is, in a sense, composed of ragas. While harmony, or the relationship of notes played simultaneously, has dominated Western music, ragas dominate Indian music. Ragas emphasize the relationship between *successive* notes. Ragas are essentially melodic music; ethnomusicologists consider them to be one of the world's most sophisticated musical expressions.

Furthermore, ragas help create what I call "vertical" music. By this I mean that ragas are internal, drawing one inward. Like the Eastern culture and religion, it is introverted. Eastern religions advocate looking within to discover the inner reality and mystery of one's being and Eastern music facilitates this process. Western music, on the other hand, is essentially "horizontal" in character. It has an intrinsic expansive quality that, by its very nature, causes it to move outward. This is typical of the Western culture, which is basically extroverted. Western religion, particularly Christianity, primarily advocates going outside oneself, toward one's fellow human beings.[13] Are we not meant to feel a burning desire to help others after a Christian worship service? Western music generally facilitates this outgoing process.*

The Mantras within the Raga

Ragas are comprised of the mantric syllables SA, RI, GA, MA, PA, DA, NI, and SA — which correspond to the DO, RE, MI, FA, SO, LA, TI, DO of Western music. These mantric syllables are sacred for the

* There are of course many exceptions to this generalization. The music of Bach is an excellent example of western music that draws us inward.

Indian musician. Each note of the raga is associated with a deity rich in symbolic meaning and mythology.

For example, the note SA — the equivalent of DO in Western music — is derived from the first name of the deity known as *Shadja Swara Daivatha*. The grandmother of all notes, she is said to have a plump body. Her complexion is red, like the lotus — a flower that demonstrates how beauty can bloom in the muddiest of waters, symbolizing the fact that even the most twisted mind can be awakened to truth. The deity Shadja has four faces that represent the four cardinal directions, and eight hands, showing that all the other notes spring from her. Her two legs, stretched out on either end of the octave, continually give birth to her endless creativity. She is dressed in white to represent her infinite purity, and in the center of her forehead is the red mark of the goddess, a sign that she is feminine and married. Riding her vehicle, the swan (also a symbol of spiritual purity), she carries a sword, which represents discernment. Shadja Swara Daivatha belongs to the race of the *Gandharvas,* a mythical community of spiritual musicians who dwell in the heavens. It is said that *Agni,* the God of fire, was the first to discover her sacred presence. Since Agni is the principal deity of the Gods and the supreme messenger between the human and the Divine, this denotes the ancient supremacy of the fundamental note SA. All the other notes in the octave are described just as richly for the Indian musician.[14]

You may recall that the word for "note" in Indian music is "swara," meaning "that which makes its own sweetness." In music, sweetness is harmony or consonance, and each note (in relationship to the fundamental) has intrinsic properties that generate healing, wholeness, and love. The fundamental note on either end of the octave is the maternal syllable SA. The fifth note, PA — a note of great stability located in the middle of the octave — is the father. The other notes are the progeny of these two. In India, there is a well-known saying: "Mata, Pita, Guru, Deivam," or "The Divine is mother, father, and teacher." This trinity parallels the musical octave.

As you might guess, the notes and deities of the musical octave are also related to the chakras: SA to the root, RI to the second chakra, GA to the abdomen, MA to the heart, PA to the throat (the creative, expressive center), DA to the third eye, and NI to the crown. The techniques of Indian music, which use these syllables in performance and composition, awaken energy in the chakras, channeling energy toward its highest fulfillment in the Divine and transforming negative energy into a positive force. In this sense, the Nada Yoga practice involving the notes of the octave actually becomes a Shakti Yoga practice that works with the chakras. Ascending and descending the musical scale simultaneously causes our awareness to ascend and descend the spine, vibrating every cell along its path and activating groups of nerves that send healing impulses to the brain and the rest of the body.

SOUNDING THE CHAKRAS

WHILE MANY BOOKS on the chakras equate a specific musical note with each chakra, usually configuring them to the major scale — C, D, E, F, G, A, B, C — it is important to recognize that this approach does not take into consideration such significant factors as the time of day or the practitioner's mood, body type, vocal range, or emotional state. Someone with a smaller or lighter body might find the key of E or G more appropriate.

One must also take into consideration the fact that the key of C contains twelve intervals, and each one of these intervals could start a new octave sequence. If you start on middle C as the fundamental, then from middle C to high C (twice the frequency) is one octave. The minor second — middle C# to high C# — offers another octave sequence, and so on. On a piano that has seven sets of C octaves, you have seven times twelve, or eighty-four keys, representing the seven sets of the twelve frequencies located with each of the seven C octaves. The individual human voice functions within a limited range, which is why choral music is so stimulating; it is made up of different vocal timbres functioning in various octave ranges that produce a wide spectrum of musical frequencies, all sounding harmoniously together.

Then there is the gender of the raga. In Indian music, ragas can be either masculine or feminine. Some are particularly powerful at certain times of the day or night, while others can be used at any time. Some ragas are seasonal and, like certain types of food, are best used during the appropriate time of the year. All this must be considered in order to achieve a more targeted effectiveness of raga and swara upon our spiritual consciousness and its development through the chakras. A vocabulary of ragas and vocal nuance also must be developed for the greatest amount of control during a session. Obviously, this level of expertise is only necessary for the highly advanced practitioner or healer. For most practical purposes, a few interval sequences are more than sufficient to keep the yogi's chakras in alignment and balance. I offer the model I follow in appendix four.

As you can see, working with the chakras through ragas and music can become incredibly detailed, but here are some rough guidelines to help you keep it simple. We already discussed the fact that low tones are harmonious with denser structures because they have slower-moving oscillations. Similarly, high tones, with their rapid wave frequency, affect subtler regions. In the same way, vowels open up a specific region to prolonged energy supply, while consonants literally hammer and chisel away at the outmoded energy structures in a chakra. Listen to any vocal rendering of classical Indian music, and you will both hear and experience this combination of vowels and consonants in the use of raga. The combination of low and high tones, together with consonants and vowels applied in a specific sequence of musical intervals, activates and opens the chakras in amazing ways. Also, when you skip over an interval or two, it causes energy to push through several chakras; this technique generates a strong force-field that helps move energy out of a particular blocked center.

In these ways, ragas can be used for a wide variety of purposes. They can help a person deal with anger, pain, jealousy, depression, frustration, or emptiness. I believe that ragas, applied in clinical settings, offer powerful therapeutic tools to treat a wide range of illnesses. As music therapy evolves, the use of melodic sequences — particularly the amazing array of possibilities found in Indian music — can be documented for their healing properties.

RHYTHM AND ENTRAINMENT

Finally, we must understand and use the musical element of rhythm in our chanting of mantras and in our breathing. Rhythmic patterns cause entrainment — the tendency for two oscillating bodies to come into phase with each other so that they vibrate together. I mentioned earlier the example of two heart-muscle cells vibrating together when brought into close proximity, or menstrual cycles that synchronize when women live in community. Entrainment produces synergy, which is the working together of two or more things or people to generate an effect greater than their individual capabilities combined. In Nada Yoga, the combined action of sound and breath produces such synergy. Another interesting parallel is that in medicine, synergy is the phenomenon whereby the combined action of two things — for example, drugs and muscles — is greater than the sum of their individual effects.

Music can be performed with or without rhythm. Chanting, no matter how slow, is often naturally rhythmic because the phrases and patterns are repeated in cycles. This is why group chanting is such a powerful phenomenon; the combined effect is far greater than that of any individual in the group. Similarly, when you chant along with a good recording, you have the same effect of entrainment. The cells, muscles, and tissues in your body are energized by the results. Boston scientist William Condon has shown that entrainment also takes place when two people have a good conversation; suddenly, their brain waves begin to oscillate synchronously.[15]

George Leonard, in his book *The Silent Pulse,* writes: "Meditation is a means for us to become more sensitive to our inner vibrations and rhythms. It may also be a means to facilitate entrainment, to tune our vibrations so that we are more 'in sync' with our world and with the people around us."[16]

PART 4

PRACTICE

THE ELEMENTS OF SOUND YOGA

The creator made the senses to flow outward-going; they go to the world of matter outside, not to the spirit within. But those sages who seek immortality look within and discover their own soul.

Katha Upanishad

CHAPTER 11

PREPARATION AND MANTRA SHASTRA

The ancients saw the world as made up of five elements: earth, water, fire, air, and space. Similarly, I have broken the practice of the Yoga of Sound into five basic components: posture, breath, sound, movement, and consciousness. We will explore each of these five elements in the chapters that follow. First, proper preparation, combined with certain observances, will help you greatly in your Yoga of Sound practice; that is the subject of this chapter.

TIME OF DAY

The Hindu tradition holds three periods of day as conducive to yoga practice. The first two are sunrise and sunset; the third is the predawn hour. At dawn and dusk, with the merging of light and darkness, nature herself is in a yogic, meditative state. As night meets day, and day meets night, everything associated with these opposites merges into the ecstasy of yogic union: male and female, intuition and reason, hot and cold — all of these are in balance. We need only tune in. When we do, our cells begin to vibrate in sympathy with nature's processes, and every part of our being becomes drawn into this prayer of yoga.

Hindus call certain mantras, yogic practices, and rituals performed at dawn and dusk *Sandhya Vandhana*. "Sandhya" means "to merge." The same term is used in Sanskrit grammar to describe the merging of two or more consonants, an obvious connection between sound and yoga.

The first three Vedic mantras provided in appendix one constitute an excellent Sandhya Vandhana practice.

The word "vandhana" means "to give praise." At dawn, the rising of the sun and the gentle stirrings of nature awaken our energy and fill us with warmth. At dusk, the changing colors of the sky and the quieting of natural activity inspire a peace that draws us into the core of our being. For those of us who live secular lives, often beginning our day with resistance or anticipation of stress and returning home burdened with financial concerns or bruised from a rough day at work, it is good to enjoy nature's help.

Another special time for prayer is the period preceding dawn. Known as the "nectar period," this is considered one of the most auspicious times for yoga and meditation. Chemically and biologically, during this period between approximately 3:00 and 4:30 in the morning, a change takes place in hormonal and neurotransmitter secretions governed by the pituitary. Hormonal secretions shift from sleep-inducing melatonin to stress-inducing cortisol and serotonin. If this changing of the guard isn't smooth, our emotions for that day can easily fall out of balance.[1] Practicing yoga during this time, especially with chanting, helps smooth the transition.

The predawn hour is also coveted by yogis because of the purity of consciousness that manifests in the air at this time. Karmic impressions are almost negligible during this period, and there is a clarity of perception that is difficult to encounter at other times of day; it is akin to starting out with a clean slate.

If practicing yoga at dawn, dusk, or the predawn hour isn't convenient for you, any time of day will suffice. But a dedicated time period is best. When you are developing a new component of your spiritual life, it is always good to set aside a special time, at least once a day, for your practice. Twice a day is even better. When we become accustomed to having a cup of coffee or a meal at a certain time of day, we naturally crave it when the hour arrives. It is the same with spiritual practice. Once we establish a habit for spiritual consciousness, we crave its undisturbed peace of mind. During this period, we find ourselves setting aside falsehoods and pretenses with natural ease and detachment. Our bodies, with their circadian rhythms, function like clocks. Being disciplined about the time of day for our practice, therefore, helps establish new grooves in our complex human mechanisms. Once established, it then becomes easy to access these grooves at any hour.

DURATION OF YOGA PRACTICE AND NUMBER OF MANTRA RECITATIONS

YOU MUST INVEST a reasonable amount of time in each of your mantra practices in order to absorb them. Once your body has learned and assimilated the effects of certain mantras, you can relinquish much of the conscious learning process and settle more deeply into the experience of yoga by employing breath control, yoga mudras, and movements either simultaneously or in sequential flow with your mantra practice.

Numbers have always played an important role in Hinduism, and most numbers have cosmological significance. The number twenty-one, for example, is considered especially significant in spiritual practice. The number three symbolizes wholeness (which comes from "holiness"), for example the many holy trinities. And the number seven represents perfection in differentiation; the seven chakras are a good example. So multiplying seven by three denotes a completeness that takes all the levels of consciousness into consideration. Hence, the optimal duration of spiritual practice is roughly twenty-one minutes. From the practical standpoint, this allows enough time to settle in, do your practice, and make a smooth return to regular activity.

When working with a particular mantra for a specific purpose, pick a certain number of days during which you will recite the mantra. During this period, say the mantra as often as possible. Alternatively, determine a set number of recitations to do every day. It is considered particularly effective to perform 108 recitations, especially with the Gayatri mantra. Other frequently used configurations are three days, seven days, and twenty-one days. Various teachers, schools, and subtraditions recommend other combinations, such as twenty, twenty-four, forty, or forty-eight days for certain mantras. This depends on the deity being invoked or the specific power desired from the chanting. I do not advise this level of detail for the general practitioner since particular rituals, dietary obligations, and restrictions apply within these contexts.

CREATING AN ENVIRONMENT FOR SPIRITUAL PRACTICE

Our environment, particularly our immediate surroundings, is crucial to effective yoga and meditation practice. In our sterile, tightly controlled, synthetic world, we are generally out of touch with nature. We get so accustomed to our artificial environments that we sometimes forget how unhealthy they are for us. This is why we need retreat facilities, monasteries, and meditation centers to constantly renew our spiritual practice. But, for most of us, our spiritual practice takes place in the heart of our lives, where we live every day.

Because carving out a practice in the midst of our lives is difficult, we need to designate a physical location for our sessions, just as we allocate specific times for our practice. This location, to which we return at the same hour every day, develops energy around it. Each time we return to this spot and harmonize our energies with those of our environment, we fortify this energy field as well as our own, which then becomes stronger and stronger with the spiritual vibrations generated by our practice. The *Bhagavad Gita* says:

> *Day after day, let the yogi continually seek the harmony of the soul by mastering the mind in a secret place, in deep solitude, hoping for nothing, desiring nothing. When the mind of the yogi is in harmony and finds rest in the Spirit within, her soul is like a lamp whose light is steady, for it burns in a shelter where no winds come.*[2]

Ideally, you will dedicate a small portion of your home to your Yoga of Sound practice — say four feet by ten feet. In the Hindu tradition, the northeast corner of the home or room is used for this purpose. It is called the *devatharchanam,* a place for honoring Divinity. This designated space serves to remind you of a space within yourself, unperturbed by the disturbances of the outer world. It is your sanctuary, into which you can direct all your processes toward their deepest resolution and fulfillment. As time goes by, this space will establish itself inside you, and you will become less dependent on the external space you initially created. It is this inner space that becomes your refuge at all times and in all places.

To make nature a greater part of our space, houseplants are excellent companions for yoga and meditation. Quiet fountains can help if you are living in a busy neighborhood or in the heart of the city. Good ventilation, cleanliness, and orderliness will greatly assist with your meditation and breathing.

Lamps, candles, icons, statues, and well-crafted artwork depicting gods or goddesses may be placed around the room for ambience. Stone, brass, or wood are recommended; stay away from synthetic materials.

HARMONY AND ATTUNEMENT

Sound is the most important factor in our practice, and we need to stay attuned to all its forms. What if we begin our practice and a neighbor starts using his lawn mower, or the garbage truck is operating outside? These distractions make gliding smoothly into the depths of our being difficult. Each time we are pulled out of our spiritual process, it will leave us fragmented. You can minimize distractions by turning off the telephone and turning down the answering machine. But if the time you have set apart for your practice is frequently infringed upon by external conditions that you cannot control, consider changing the time frame. Remember, our sensitivities become heightened many times over during Sound Yoga practices; we don't want to spend most of our time fighting off disturbances.

If noise is a constant problem, headphones can be an asset, especially the noise-canceling type created by Bose or Sennheiser; these special headphones can filter out a lot of unpleasant frequencies, but they are also expensive. When necessary, I recommend that you use regular headphones to create a pleasant inner space with sacred music or nature sounds; use them only when you really can't concentrate on your practice, because headphones cut you off from experiencing and working with the natural energy of your environment. Also, never use headphones when singing along with a CD, as it will affect the accuracy of your pitch. In general, I recommend a good, high-fidelity stereo system or boom box for playing cassettes and CDs to help in your Sound Yoga practice.

Ultimately, the best response to intrusive sounds is to include them in your practice; exclude nothing. Instead of judging the sounds or wishing they weren't happening, accept them. Relax and observe their effects on your body. You will experience sensations and even visual manifestations as the sounds trigger energy movements in you. Breathe slowly, deeply, and audibly. Practice Brahmari Mudra (appendix four) if the noise is unbearable. Offer minimum resistance to the sound, and it will pass right through you. The more you resist it — especially mentally — the more your body will experience discomfort. Learn to allow your body to become permeable, like a transparent membrane. Visualize the sound waves passing through you and out of you. Become aware of spaciousness beyond the sound. Attune yourself to that vibration, rather than to how the sound affects you; this way, you will experience tremendous freedom and power.

DIET

THIS MAY BE OBVIOUS, but I remind my students that we are what we eat. The vibrations of our food become the substance of our bodies and our minds. This is why mass-produced meat products, which result from subjecting livestock to unnatural conditions and inhumane treatment, are not ideal for the yogic lifestyle. If you eat meat, try to get organic meats without any genetically modified ingredients.

Don Campbell, in his book *The Mozart Effect,* cites a study conducted at the West Virginia University School of Medicine. Based on closely observing more than 1,400 persons with inner-ear problems, the researchers concluded that hearing significantly improved in those who were given nutritional counseling and put on diets low in saturated fat, simple sugars, and table salt, and high in whole-grain cereals, vegetables, and fresh fruits.[3]

Following the yogic method of eating, I recommend reserving half your stomach for solid foods and one-fourth for liquids, leaving one-fourth free for air. This can be applied to all your meals, or at least two out of three.

Also, observe the coincidence between food consumption and the tone and clarity of your vocal expressions. You may find that minimizing consumption of dairy products frees your vocal expression immensely.

MANTRA SHASTRA

FINALLY, the ancient texts detail many guidelines for proper and effective yoga practice. I have augmented these guidelines with further ideas I've discovered through my own practice:

- Cleanse your body before beginning your Yoga of Sound practice; a shower is ideal. If you have showered recently, brush your teeth, or at least rinse your mouth three times with water. If an hour or two has passed since you showered, a quick wash of the face, hands, and feet is also highly recommended.
- When showering to prepare for your Yoga of Sound practice, shower consciously, mentally purifying your body, mind, and heart as the water washes over you. Join your palms in reverence at least once during your shower to invoke a sense of the sacred in your body.
- Wear simple, loose, comfortable clothing. Cotton, silk, and wool are good conductors of yogic energy.
- Light a stick of incense to create a sacred atmosphere in your dedicated yoga practice area. Smell is associated with the root chakra and can help connect our awareness to the presence of spirit in matter.
- Offer a flower or fruit to an image of the Divine that adorns your altar. This immediately places your practice in a larger sacred context.
- Sprinkle some water around your meditation seat or yoga mat, symbolically purifying your space and cleansing it of negative energy.
- Face east or north. These directions are traditionally considered most powerful for mantra recitation.
- Try to do your practice before meals. The process of digestion requires energy that should not be diverted from yogic pursuits.
- Perform a fixed number of recitations by using a set of mantra beads, or decide on a fixed amount of time for chanting a specific mantra.
- Use an asana, or yoga pose, with your mantra. Ideally, you will maintain the same pose for the duration of chanting a specific mantra.

- If you are using movement while chanting, keep your awareness centered in your body and your physical sensations.
- Try not to allow your eyes to wander. Keep them fixed on your altar or a scene of natural beauty outside your window, or close your eyes and choose a center of reference in your body.
- Vary your internal center of reference among the navel, the heart, and the head so that you can work with at least three distinct vibratory energies.
- Vary your chanting between the loud external repetitions, whispering the mantra on your breath, and sounding it internally. These dynamics will help awaken a wide spectrum of consciousness.
- Try to do your practice at predetermined times, at least once or twice each day. If you miss these times for any reason, make it up somehow, even if only for a shorter period.
- Try to maintain solitude while you do your practice. If people are around, avoid speech during your practice; it will drain away the energy generated by your mantra.
- Chant with intense devotion so that the process takes you into your depths.
- Use a notebook to keep track of your recitations and to make journal entries relating to your experiences. See "Fortifying Your Practice Year-Round" in chapter seventeen.
- At the end of your recitation, spend a few minutes to become aware of what the mantra has revealed. It may be an insight into a problem, a sense of peace, a resolution to a situation, a vision of spiritual beauty, a palpable feeling of intense joy, increased energy, a sense of well-being, or a profound awareness of the Divine presence. Appreciate and offer thanks for this revelation each time, whatever it may be.

CHANTING WITHOUT CEASING

Jesus' injunction to "pray without ceasing" was taken to heart by the monks and mystics of Christianity. They, too, used mantras such as the name of Jesus, the phrase "Lord, have Mercy on me," or *Maranatha,* which in Aramaic — the language Jesus spoke — means "Come, Lord." An interesting anagram of this word is *Ramanatha,* which means "Lord Rama" for the Hindu. The devoted Sound yogi is also dedicated to chanting all the time, not only for him or herself, but for others, for the world, for people in need, for cultures in crisis.

The whole purpose of mantra shastra — the optimal times of day for chanting, suggestions for maintaining a sacred environment, appropriate diet, and so on — is to enable us to create a field of energy strong enough to allow the power of our prayers and intentions to affect our lives and the world. This becomes possible only when our energy is continually renewed through spiritual practice, because this same field can easily become depleted by life situations. It is the power of accumulation that helps us build a reservoir of spiritual energy in our body, our mind, and our heart. We then share this refined quality of energy with others through our relationships, our professions, and our acts of kindness in the world, all of which contribute to making our world a better place for everyone.

CHAPTER 12

POSTURE

Proper posture, which invariably implies proper symmetry, generates the optimal distribution of the spiritual and physiological effects of our Yoga of Sound practice, because underlying the symmetry of our posture are harmonic proportions — the same proportions that allow us to appreciate beauty in music.

A beautiful image from Christianity compares the body to a temple for the Holy Spirit. I like to say that, because temples and cathedrals have wonderful acoustics, this analogy is particularly significant in Sound Yoga. Interestingly, this image is more than metaphorical, as demonstrated by studying the golden mean.

THE GOLDEN MEAN

THE GOLDEN MEAN — also known as the golden section, golden ratio, or Divine proportion — is a harmonic proportion that inspires us to identify with much of the beauty in art, nature, and the human body. The proportions of harmony, in other words, generate beauty. A well-proportioned body is beautiful because it is musical and dominated by the golden section.

The golden section is a ratio or proportion of 1 to 1.618033-988749895..., which is designated by the Greek letter *phi*. It can be derived via a number of geometric constructions, each of which divides a line segment at the unique point where the ratio of the whole line (A) to the large segment (B) is the same as the ratio of the large segment (B) to the small segment (C). In other words, A is to B as B is to C. This occurs only where A is phi times B and B is phi times C.*

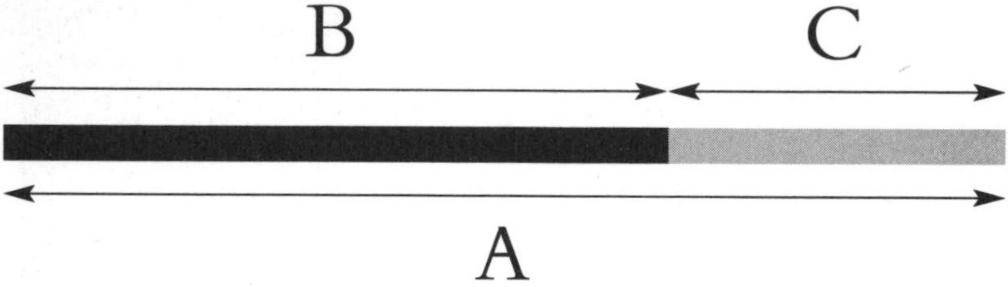

This ratio has been used by humans for millennia; the Egyptians incorporated it in the design of their pyramids. The Greeks, too, were familiar with this ratio, and used it to create beauty and balance in their architecture. Plato considered it to be "the most binding of all mathematical relationships, and the key to the physics of the universe."

Renaissance artists, such as Leonardo da Vinci, knew this ratio as the Divine proportion, and they used it to create beauty and balance in their artwork; da Vinci's painting *The Last Supper* is a key example. The Cathedral of Notre Dame in Paris was built using this proportion, which continues to appear throughout modern architecture, for example in the United Nations building in New York.

The golden mean is also found in the Bible, in the design of Noah's ark, the Ark of the Covenant, and the colors of the Tabernacle. It appears throughout mathematics, in the shape of the earth, in plant spirals, in our DNA, in the solar system, in the shapes of dolphins and butterflies, and even in the behavior of the stock market.

The golden mean is still being discovered in numerous ancient cathedrals, temples, and mosques. With the spectacular acoustics in such places, sound not only carries clearly to every corner of the edifice, but seems to come alive with an otherworldly spirit. These structures

* For a thorough understanding of phi and the golden mean, visit http://goldennumber.net, a fabulous Website created by Gary Meisner.

were built to remind human beings of a supreme intelligence and power that was the source of their being. To enter such a holy place created a sense of awe, as though one were in the very bowels of the infinite.

For our purposes, the important occurrences of the golden mean are in music and in the proportions of the human body. The golden mean can be seen in the entire length of the human body, in the hand, and in the face. It has been found that a face that lacks the proportions of the golden mean results in health problems that can be rectified by orthodontic appliances. As an interesting corollary, the shape of the human ear is based on the golden mean, and so are the proportions of human teeth, both associated with sound, speech, and listening.

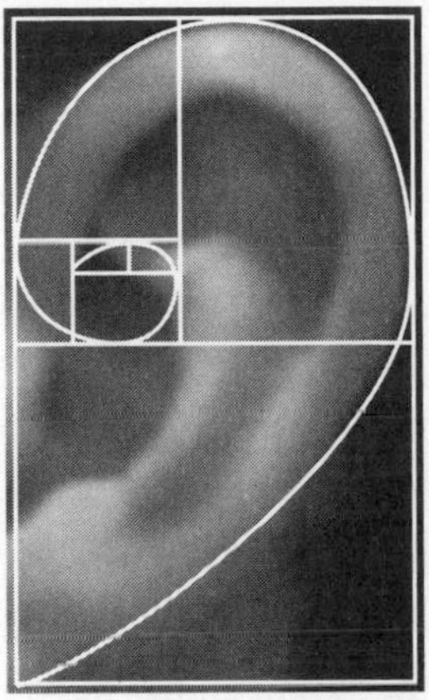

Musically, the tempered intervals listed in chapter ten are based on this Divine proportion. What is more, climaxes in musical compositions are often found to occur in a time sequence proportionate to the golden mean, at roughly the phi point (61.8 percent of the way through the piece). Mozart's sonatas and Beethoven's Fifth Symphony demonstrate this, as does music from Bartók, Debussy, Schubert, Bach, and Satie. Key points in human aging and development, from gestation to old age, also occur in this Divine proportion. Reproductive processes in multicellular organisms follow this proportion so accurately that urban population growth can be predicted using it.

Joachim-Ernst Berendt cites German scholar Thomas Michael Schmidt on the prevalence of the golden mean in relation to the human body as follows:

> *"The navel divides the entire body length in the proportions of the golden section . . . The nipples divide the entire width of the human body with stretched arms in the proportions of the golden section . . . The knee divides the entire leg in the proportions of the golden section . . . The eyebrows divide the head in the proportion of the golden section . . . The elbow joint divides the entire arm including*

> *the hand in the proportions of the golden section... Inasmuch as the human body is structured by the golden section — by musical proportion, that is — one can call it a sounding work of art because its shape is dominated by the most perfect mathematical proportions. Thus it is entirely correct to say that, at least in terms of... anatomy, the [human] is meant to be perfect."*[1]

It is precisely these proportions in our body that allow us to appreciate music and distinguish among noise, bad music, good music, and sublime music.

THE TEMPLE OF THE SOUL

Once we understand the natural harmonies between our bodies and music, we can use our voice to give praise inside the temple of the human body and summon the energy of the infinite into this sacred space. When we turn our gaze to our interior and observe the abysmal darkness inside us, we realize that the body is not a solid structure, but an intense field of vibration with an infinite depth of resonance. This awareness allows us to sense the presence and substance of the soul. An oft-quoted statement from the German mystic Meister Eckhart sums this up eloquently: "Think not that the soul is in the body," he says, "but rather that the body is in the soul."[2]

Conventional Western postures of prayer represent attitudes and qualities of the heart that determine the relationship between our own soul and Spirit. Kneeling, for example, is a sign of humility — a visible submission to God's greatness, and an acknowledgment of our need to align in loving relationship with this greatness. In the yoga tradition, posture is associated with the stabilization and flow of energy. By combining East and West — energy distribution and attitude of the soul — in our practice of the Yoga of Sound, we can create the ideal conditions for our inner journey.

In the East, calmness of the body is known to create calmness in the mind. This allows the yogi to prolong the period of meditation in comfort. Calmness allows us to view the very nature of the mind, rather than being preoccupied with the varying phenomena — the "mind stuff" constantly arising within the mind field. As I mentioned before, Patanjali's opening yoga sutra states that yoga is *"chitta vritti nirodha* — the cessation of the modifications of the mind." When the flux subsides, the mind functions as a well-polished lens, through which we can gaze into the depths of the soul.

Proper posture also aids concentration, which is the ability of the mind to focus on a specific area with only one thought flowing continuously toward that single reference point. In order to sustain this one-pointed concentration with a minimum of interference from mental distractions, the body literally holds the mind in check by virtue of its own steadiness. Posture is therefore essential to creating the optimal conditions for yoga.

In the West, posture is first used to acknowledge the presence of God, and then to bring the self — the ego — into that presence. In the East, the process is reversed, beginning with the self and then expanding into the conscious realization of the Divine essence. Both approaches have the same objective. The yogic approach is especially important for us today because we often lack body consciousness. Most of our day is spent at a computer or in a car. Our minds, too, are furiously racing around, and dragging our bodies along for the ride. When our consciousness is awakened through proper posture, we notice a significant difference in our body-mind relationship.

At the outset of your practice, therefore, the first step is to determine where you are in relationship with your body. By bringing body and soul into harmony, you can gauge your relationship with the natural world and with the Divine. Samadhi, as we know, should include all levels and dimensions. Take a few moments at the start of your practice to become aware of your mental, physical, psychological, and spiritual condition. If you have been living the past few minutes, hours, days, or months disconnected from your body, you will know it. If you have gotten locked into a state of pride or arrogance, you will know it. If you are disturbed on some level of your being, you will know it. Based on this information, you can adopt a posture that helps restore balance and facilitates healing in these relationships.

Posture also provides us with stability and strength. Our spiritual practice should be built on a strong foundation that we can fall back on with trust. As we delve into our depths, we can then do so in the comfort of knowing that when we return to everyday consciousness, a secure home awaits us in our body.

The rich will make temples for Shiva.
What shall I, a poor man, do?
My legs are pillars,
The body the shrine,
The head a cupola of gold.
Listen, Oh Lord of the meeting rivers,
Things standing shall fall,
But the moving shall ever stay.

Basavanna, 820 B.C.[3]

THE BASIC POSTURES

MOST OF THE ASANAS of Hatha Yoga offer variations of how to stand, sit, or lie down. In the following exercises, I will introduce you to these three basic options, and offer you simple meditations involving all the elements of Sound Yoga. I will leave the twisting and bending to the expert Hatha Yoga teachers.

Lying Down

LYING DOWN on the floor is known as *savasana,* the corpse pose. Despite its dismal name, this is an important posture; we can use it not only to relax the body in preparation for our practices, but also to distribute the flow of energy generated by a single practice, a series of practices, or at the end of a session. The corpse pose is also ideal for deep listening meditations.

The Method

1. Lie flat on your back on a yoga mat, rug, or blanket. Stretch your legs out in front of you in a straight line. Briefly place your feet together to align your body symmetrically, then let them go slack. With your arms beside you on the floor, keep your hands slightly away from your body and facing upward. Relax your whole body and allow all your body energies to sink into the ground. When your body has attained

some equilibrium, focus your attention on the movement of your abdomen as your body breathes at its own natural pace. As you focus on this simple movement, allow your body to become more and more relaxed. This is *savasana.* Now you will begin your Yoga of Sound meditation in this posture.

2. As you attune to your breath, introduce the mantra *so-ham,* using the syllable *so* on the inhalation and *ham* on the exhalation. The meaning of this mantra is simply "I am," similar to the answer Moses received when he asked who was appearing to him through the burning bush. The *so-ham* mantra helps us enter the ground of our being, which my mentor Bede Griffiths describes as being present everywhere, in everything, yet always escaping our grasp. "It is the 'ground' of all existence," he explained, "that from which all things come, and to which all things return, but which itself never appears."[4]

Don't underestimate the simplicity of the corpse pose. Famous South Indian mystic Ramana Maharshi had his spiritual awakening when he lay down on the floor one day and imitated his death in this position. The corpse pose expresses a depth of surrender and facilitates profound healing as we allow ourselves to be received into the earth's bosom, merging our own energies with her force of gravity and returning to the ground of our being. In the spirit of the Upanishads, "The wise should surrender speech in the mind, the mind in the knowing self, the knowing self in the spirit of the universe, and the spirit of the universe in the spirit of peace."[5]

In preparing for our Yoga of Sound practice, it is good to begin with an act of surrender that relinquishes our personal agendas and any preconceived notions of what our experience should be.

Standing

Standing in *praarthanaasana** — the posture of prayer — is an amazing and wonderful method of balancing our energy. One advantage of this posture is that you can practice it almost anywhere — in a bathroom,

---

* *Praarthana* means "prayer."

or even a closet. It is particularly helpful if you need a moment to gather yourself or relieve tension during office hours.

The Method

1. Stand in an upright position, with feet together and palms joined at the heart in the *namaste* gesture; fingertips are touching lightly but the palms are slightly apart with space between the fingers of each hand. This is known as *anjali mudra*. Close your eyes, relax your face, and breathe evenly. Particularly relax your shoulders, and allow each section of your body to consciously relax, beginning with the top of your head and proceeding down toward your feet. In doing this, you are not only relaxing each section of your body along the proportions of the golden mean (since so much of the body is proportioned according to this ratio), but you are allowing the energies of each of these sections to flow downward into the earth, helping ground your consciousness in a place of depth. Rest for some time on the soles of your feet and experience the subtle shifts in balance from one foot to the other as your body naturally adjusts to hold the position. This awareness gently stimulates ida and pingala, the hot and cold spiritual meridians on either side of the body.

2. Draw your awareness into your heart-space, and follow the natural breath process in this region. If you find that your mind is distracted or uncoordinated, use your nostrils to breathe slowly and deliberately into your heart space, but keep your mouth closed. When exhaling, slowly release the breath through your mouth with a gentle "aah" sound. Regulate your exhalation in your throat so that the sound is not as pronounced as in regular speech, but more like an ocean wave — a soothing sound that releases tension and calms the entire nervous system. If you perceive emotional unrest in your body, you may exhale with a few throaty groans or sighs; follow these with a few ocean-wave "aahs."

3. If unrest continues, exhale slowly and ride the sound "aah" on your breath, as though you were whispering it into the space in front of you. Allow your palms to move apart slowly and make room for your breath, allowing the winds of heaven to blow through them. Keep your fingertips facing skyward, the fingers slightly erect and comfortably apart. Separate your palms until they are comfortably at, or slightly beyond, your shoulder blades. If your discomfort is extreme, spread your palms wide apart to dissipate the energy. Be mindful of the energy between your palms as you work your breath and match your hand movements with the expansion of your lungs. Notice the emotional quality of your heart-space being transformed. "Open wide ancient doors; let him enter, the King of glory."[6]

   Inhale, breathing slowly and deeply into your heart space, as you bring your palms together at your heart in perfect synchrony with your breath. As your palms move closer together, it will feel as if you are compacting your breath. Consciously assimilate this compressed energy into your heart-space, then allow it to expand as you exhale. Work this contraction and expansion until you feel that you've eliminated all the tension you've been trying to release.

   This repetition should replicate a musical performance on an accordion, filmed in slow motion. Your mindfulness packs presence and punch into the practice. Slowly resolve the movement to a place of stillness, your hands returning to the namaste gesture and pressing gently against your solar plexus. Breathe naturally and stay relaxed in this position for a short while, keenly aware of the spaciousness and depth created by the movement. Remain alert for any subtle sensations or movements that may register in your body awareness.

You will find that this practice helps release emotional buildup, such as after a tense business meeting or a heated conversation with a loved one.

Sitting

There are three ways to sit for your Sound Yoga practice: cross-legged, between your heels, and on a chair. Having a woolen blanket or rug on the floor underneath you helps your practice feel more grounded. Meditation practices produce such a subtle quality of consciousness that it is necessary to balance this with a connection to the earth's energy. This "grounding" makes it easier for us to continue with regular activities after our spiritual exercises.

If even *sukhasana,* the easiest version of the cross-legged posture, feels difficult, try sitting between your heels or using a prayer stool. As a last alternative, use a chair; this is a wiser choice than using an uncomfortable posture that generates improper flow of energy in the body.

One last word of advice: Please do not use your designated time for spiritual practice to develop flexibility in your legs or aim toward the ideal posture; this should be done at another time. Try to finish your stretches and muscle toning before you engage in Yoga of Sound practices.

Sitting Cross-Legged

This Eastern way of sitting is difficult for many Westerners — sometimes even impossible, but there are many preparatory yoga stretches that can help make your legs more supple and allow for a more comfortable cross-legged posture. Your local Hatha Yoga teacher can help you achieve this.

Having researched postures for thousands of years, yogis claim that sitting cross-legged is the most conducive to the flow of life force (prana). This is because the base of the spine and the two points represented by the knees pressing toward the ground form a holy triangle that naturally collects and concentrates our body energies. Second, since the legs correspond to all pairs of opposites — male and female, rational and intuitive, hot and cold — their interlocking facilitates an inner harmony between these pairs.

The full-lotus posture is an advanced asana. It is not recommended for your practice of Sound Yoga unless you are extremely flexible in your legs or you are an advanced Hatha Yoga practitioner. Because of the damage you can do yourself through inexperienced application, the lotus posture has been deliberately omitted from this section.

The following are variations on the cross-legged posture. Choose what is most comfortable for you, and work with that position until you can naturally move on to the next. Don't force a position; it is not worth sitting uncomfortably for your Sound Yoga practices. Be patient and allow your comfort level to evolve organically as you gain experience. There are two important guidelines:

1. Whichever cross-legged posture you adopt, be sure that your knees are at, or below, the level of your hips — never above them. A good indication of an imbalanced posture is that your knees will start to rise, or that your body wants to lean forward to restore balance. If necessary, use a cushion to raise your hips higher than your knees; it will give you the stability you need.
2. It is not a good idea to lean on a backrest or against the wall because an independently erect spine is the ideal conductor for energy in the body, ensuring its optimal distribution throughout our nervous system. If you have a spinal problem, consult with an experienced yoga instructor or physiotherapist. As you ease into the posture, you must be able to hold your upper body erect and relaxed; your abdomen should sit comfortably into your hips; and you should be able to relax your face and shoulders comfortably.

The Method

SUKHASANA, THE EASY POSTURE: Sit with your legs comfortably crossed and use a cushion to raise your buttocks until you can hold your spine comfortably erect with your hips higher than your knees.

SIDDHASANA (VARIATION), THE STABLE POSTURE: Pull your left foot close to your pelvis, then pull your right foot as close as you can to the front of your left shin so that both ankles are pressed against the floor. You can do this in any order, but make sure your feet are not placed one above the other. Ideally, both knees should be pressing against the floor. Prop a cushion under your buttocks if you are unsteady when trying to straighten your spine; avoid leaning forward.

ARDHA PADMASANA, THE HALF-LOTUS: This is a compromise on the full-lotus position. Pull your left foot close to your pelvis with your left ankle pressing against the floor. Pull your right foot onto your left thigh, as close as possible to your pelvic area; it may alternatively rest on your left calf or ankle, whichever is most comfortable. You might find your right knee off the ground. If this is the case, raise your buttocks with a cushion or folded blanket so that you can lower your right knee to the ground. Try the reverse order, as well, with the right leg under the left, to see if that works better for you.

Sitting between Your Heels

VAJRASANA: This posture is excellent for the breathing practices you will learn in chapter thirteen. Yogis claim that it aids the digestive process immensely, and you might have noticed that the Japanese use it formally for dining. Sitting between your heels naturally draws your attention to the center of gravity deep in the abdomen, known as the *hara* in Japanese Zen. It's an excellent posture for centering.

The Method

KNEEL DOWN with your feet sufficiently far apart to accommodate your buttocks, then gently ease your buttocks downward until they rest comfortably in the air between your heels. Take some time to allow your lower torso and all the energies in your abdominal area to settle into your hip and buttock region. Advanced practitioners may spread their heels wide enough for the buttocks to actually touch the ground. The upper body is held in balance by the hips and the base of the spine, which must be held independently erect. Next, relax your upper torso, upper chest, and shoulders, allowing the energies in these regions to find stability and balance in the abdominal area, which in turn finds its balance in the pelvic region. Rest your palms on your thighs and ensure that your arms are relaxing at the most natural angle for your position. Once you know that your hands, arms, shoulders, and entire upper body are relaxed, begin to relax your head and face.

USING A PRAYER BENCH: If you find it difficult or painful to sit between your heels, you may use a prayer bench. This simple device allows you to sit in vajrasana without putting pressure on your heels. The bench takes all the weight of your body, leaving your heels free and relaxed.

Sitting on a Chair

YOU SHOULDN'T FEEL ashamed of sitting on a chair, as you can still derive most of the benefits offered by Sound Yoga by using one. Just remember to place the chair on a woolen rug or blanket so that you feel grounded.

The Method

THE CHAIR OR STOOL should be neither too high nor too low. Ideally, your thighs should slope downward slightly. Position your buttocks in the middle of the seat for the best balance, or move a bit closer to the edge for more spinal alertness.

ALIGNMENT AND SYMMETRY

WHATEVER YOUR POSITION, remember to check the symmetry of your body from time to time and make the necessary adjustments to maintain a natural state of balance. Verify that your weight and energy are evenly distributed throughout your body. It is natural for the body to shift its weight subtly in response to movements of energy that take place during Sound Yoga practice. Monitor these shifts, and channel your body responses with poise and grace.

Take care not to force your body into rigid postures of equilibrium — a common error among meditation practitioners. Sometimes there is a tendency to remove oneself from one's body and objectify one's posture, trying to "look good" from the outside. Tension may result. The only tension in your body should be the concentration of energy at the base of your spine and upper thighs, on either side of the genitals; this tension allows you to consciously experience and channel the subtle currents of the life force through the chakras located along the spinal cord. Consequently, if the spinal cord is not held erect and relaxed, these currents of energy may be dissipated or may fail to be channeled toward their highest potential. To simplify the process, once your body is aligned keep your head comfortably balanced; avoid stooping or looking up. Remember to constantly relax your face, shoulders, hips, and pelvis.

CHAPTER 13

THE BREATH

Next in importance after posture comes pranayama, the control of breath. Today we know that each time we inhale, life-giving oxygen is drawn into our bloodstream; each time we exhale, we rid our body of toxic carbon dioxide. But air is also primary to the experience of audible sound.

An ancient story from the Sufi tradition points to the connections between life, breath, body, and music. When the Creator fashioned the human body, the human soul refused to enter because it didn't want to take on the body's limitations. The Creator then began to play music. In order to feel the fullness of this music through the senses and receptivity of the human form, the soul was coaxed into the body. The soul continues to receive its life from the Creator by breathing in this music. Indeed, the Divine is continually replenishing our life through the music of our breath.

RHYTHM OF BREATH, RHYTHM OF LIFE

THOUSANDS OF YEARS AGO, yogis realized that the air we breathe contains prana, a force that invigorates both body and soul. This is why pranayama — the control of prana — is crucial to yoga practice. Learning to regulate this life force holds the keys to optimal health and longevity. Chanting and singing naturally require control of the breath. Conversely, control of the breath enhances our chanting and mantric practice.

Yoga, like Tai Chi and other ancient fitness practices, was developed by observing nature. Yogis noticed that creatures with rapid breathing rates, such as the hummingbird and the rabbit, had shorter life spans; creatures with slower and longer breathing rates, such as the elephant and the tortoise, lived longer. By deliberately manipulating and slowing their own breathing rates, yogis realized that they could increase their life spans, thereby extending their capacity for self-realization. In other words, the proper rhythm, another fundamental aspect of music, is essential to our health and longevity.

Inhaling Harmony, Exhaling Dissonance

YOGIS ALSO OBSERVED a direct association between breathing and emotional states. They noticed that when one is peaceful and content with life, breathing is smooth, evenly paced, and slower. Conversely, when we're emotionally upset or disturbed, our breathing is jerky, irregular, and rapid. Through experimentation, yogis realized that they could produce a state of contentment by breathing slowly, smoothly, and evenly.

Present-day microbiologist Candice Pert has found in her research that a great deal of unresolved emotional toxicity remains lodged in the upper intestine in the form of "information molecules."[1] Yogic breathing, which seeks to eliminate as much air as possible from the lungs, can help evacuate unwanted emotion from the body. The result is greater clarity and renewed energy. Despite unpleasant experiences and stressful circumstances in our lives, it is possible for us to maintain a happy and peaceful disposition by learning to work with our breath.

Proper intake of breath improves blood circulation and ensures that the blood receives the optimal amount of oxygen. Oxygen supplies the fuel for carrying out the blood's most important task: defending against diseases and assisting in the healing of wounds. The blood also helps circulate thermal energy around our body. "Breathing correctly is the key to better fitness, muscle strength, stamina, and athletic endurance," says Dr. Michael Yessis, Ph.D., a fitness writer for *Muscle and Fitness Magazine*.[2]

Proper breathing even reduces the threat of cancer; when the oxygen saturation of blood falls, conditions become ripe for the creation of cancer. Oxygen is removed from the arterial blood as it passes through the capillary system. If arterial blood is deficient in oxygen, or if the blood flow is restricted by blocked arteries, then tissues oxygenated by the latter stages of the capillary system may be so deprived of oxygen as to become cancerous.[3] Dr. Otto Warburg, in a well-known and often-quoted lecture to Nobel laureates, explains: "All carcinogens impair respiration directly or indirectly by deranging capillary circulation, a statement that is proven by the fact that no cancer cell exists without exhibiting impaired respiration. Deprive a cell of 35 percent of its oxygen for 48 hours and it may become cancerous."[4]

Most people have had their breathing checked via a stethoscope during a medical checkup. When listening to a patient's chest, doctors proceed symmetrically; first they listen to the left side, then the right side in the same region to determine if there's any difference. Even more interesting, the breathing sounds are categorized according to their location, pitch, intensity, and ratio of inspiration to expiration. Doctors actually listen to the "tone" of our breathing to determine whether we are healthy or ill; obstructions to our breathing reflect obstruction in our optimal energy flow — a point I elaborated on when discussing Shakti Yoga in chapter eight.

When there are no obstructions to the airways in our lungs, normal air movement produces normal breathing sounds. For instance, "vesicular breathing sounds," the primary normal breathing sounds, are heard throughout most of the lungs. Vesicular breathing is soft and low-pitched, with the inspiratory sounds being longer than the expiratory sounds. "Tracheal breathing sounds," on the other hand, are usually relatively high-pitched and loud. "Bronchial breathing sounds" are loud, high-pitched, and close to the surface. Finally, there are "bronchovesicular breathing sounds," which are of intermediate intensity and pitch; in this case, the inspiratory and expiratory sounds are equal in length.[5]

Obstructions in our airways, caused by such things as constriction, fluid, or hyperexpansion, result in abnormal breathing sounds. Doctors listen for abnormal sounds called "crackles," which are discontinuous, nonmusical, brief sounds heard more commonly on inspiration. When listening to crackles, doctors pay special attention to their loudness, pitch, duration, number, timing in the respiratory cycle, location, pattern from breath to breath, change after a cough, or shift in position.[6]

Any musician reading this will immediately realize that we are dealing here with pitch, intensity, and duration, the three fundamental qualities of the musical note that every student of music learns about first. This brings us to the audible breath, which is an important practice for the sound yogi.

THE AUDIBLE BREATH: THE ROAR OF THE SOUND YOGI

For the sound yogi, the audible breath serves as a lens — a magnifying glass through which we can perceive and harmonize the many layers of energy fields within our body. The breath, when made audible, also allows for greater control and manipulation of emotion. Most of all, the sound of breathing helps us contain and work with the sound of the mantra or any other sonic form of yoga. The mingling of breath and sound act as a sort of friction-stick that ignites the fire of devotion.

Hatha yogis will recognize this practice as the *ujjai* breath. As Yoga of Sound practitioners, we listen intently to the breath so that we can listen and perceive *through* the breath, even when it is almost imperceptible. This is the key to sound and silence, the contrasts of which open the doors to inner perception.

The Method

Sit in a posture that allows your body to become quiet, still, and relaxed. Breathing naturally, observe your body for a short time. You can now begin to modulate the flow of air as it passes in and out of your lungs by breathing audibly. The secret is to learn to do this with your mouth closed, meaning that you inhale and exhale through your nostrils, but sound is produced in your throat and mouth cavity as follows:

1. Inhaling: When inhaling, modulate the flow of air in your throat by a gentle contraction of the glottis, as I will describe. Slightly drop your lower jaw and allow your tongue to recede slightly into the back of your throat in your upper larynx,

pressing it against your tonsils; this process seems to "thicken" the tongue. By experimenting with your tongue, nostrils, glottis, and lower jaw, all functioning in concert, you will be able to regulate the air flowing into your lungs by controlling its passage through your throat; this will produce an audible sound. Your abdomen should be relaxed so that air can flow smoothly into the bottom of your lungs when you begin to inhale. You must also relax your upper body so that your breath can "rise" as you continue your inhalation, and so that you can feel the pressure of the air and energy against your spine as they rise.

2. Exhaling: Exhaling is similar to inhaling, but you can lessen the pressure of your tongue against the back of your throat. You may experiment with moving the tip of your tongue slightly forward, toward your teeth; this releases the pressure in your upper larynx and pushes more air into your mouth cavity, which is where you are controlling the air. While exhaling, use your abdominal muscles to gently push the air out of your lower lungs and into your mouth. Maintain a slight pressure in your throat so that the contracted glottis can regulate the outflowing air. Again, this becomes easy if you breathe audibly, producing a soft sound in your throat as you exhale. The effect is like the sound of an ocean wave. Just remember to keep your mouth closed during the process. Eventually, the sound will be produced by minimal effort and coordination of muscles.

A Learning Tool

If you are unable to figure out how to breathe audibly, you can inhale with your mouth open. The sound will happen naturally. When your lungs are partially filled with air — halfway through your inhalation — gently close your mouth and keep inhaling, while continuing to produce the same sonic effect for the rest of your in-breath. Similarly, when exhaling, begin audibly with your mouth open, then close your mouth midway during your exhalation and continue producing the sound as you complete the breath. Do this as many times as feels comfortable for you. Stop if you feel over-oxygenated; never force your body beyond its natural capacity. Once you get the principle, apply the technique without opening your mouth.

Meditation

> To deepen the experience, listen intently to the sound of your breathing. Be aware of the process by which the sound originates with your breath and then builds up during inhalation. Likewise, try to enter the energy of the sound as it diminishes during exhalation. Observe its disappearance as it tapers off into the silence of your after-breath. Rest in that silence, and through it enter into the depths of your being. Notice how the silence fills you, embraces you, and draws you into its sacred presence. Hold your breath outside yourself for a few moments, then observe the reemergence of breath and sound when you inhale in the presence of that silence. Feel the vibrations caused by your breathing coursing through your body.

THAT WHICH LINKS BODY AND SPIRIT

THE BREATH is a key element, not only in Hindu yoga practice, but in any spiritual practice, as shown in Buddhist meditation and Christian contemplative prayer. Why? Our breath is the most palpable link between the manifest reality of our physical existence and the unknown world of the spirit. When we observe the breath, we realize that it is not something we own; neither is it something we do. Rather, breathing is continually happening in us all the time. Each breath is a sign that the universe is giving us our existence at this moment. Through its contiguity, we are offered life in all its dimensions. Our breathing also gives us the totality of the present moment as an eternal now — a place from which we can be conscious that each breath is different, new — a fresh affirmation that we are receiving the gift of life.

The perspective that accompanies our breathing instills in us a sense of equality. We are not the only ones given life; that which breathes into us is, at this moment, breathing existence into every living being. The same breath has been breathed by every creature since the beginning of time, and the same breath will sustain life in all creatures yet to be born.

In this sense, there is only one breath — one life for all — making our breath a wonderfully unifying and democratic process.

BREATHING DEEPLY, CHANTING STRONGLY

To reach the full capacity of our voice, we must learn to maximize the capacity of our lungs and control the flow of our breath, especially during exhalation. We do not use the full capacity of our lungs in normal breathing; most of us take shallow breaths. When we first come into this world, we breathe deeply. Watch a baby's abdomen and you will immediately see that the lower lungs are well utilized. When we breathe deeply, we are closer to our natural state of being and to the state of yoga. Our breathing changes when we are stressed out. You will notice that fear often acts as a knot, blocking the respiratory tract and causing breathing to become shallow and irregular.

Learning how to consciously breathe into all the areas of our lungs, and how to modulate our breathing effectively, can help us cope with stressful situations and offer us clarity, peace, and renewed energy. Employing all the areas of our lungs also improves our tonal and vocal range considerably, enabling us to produce clear, beautiful pitches in our music, hold steady notes, create vocal ornamentation, and, most important of all, resolve our tones through smooth transitions. These vocal techniques have a direct effect on our consciousness, producing comparable psychological and spiritual conditions, such as single-minded concentration, harmony of being, resolution of anxiety and unwanted emotion, and the transformation of negative energy and thought patterns.

As we reach deep into the spiritual realms of consciousness, our breath functions as a bridge between the known and the unknown, the conscious and unconscious minds, the material and spiritual worlds. The following exercise will help bridge these realms.

Sectional Breathing: Divide and Rule

Having learned to regulate the flow of air in and out of your body, you are now ready to explore the various sections of the lungs that govern your functional energy fields.

The British were well known for their policy of "divide and rule," a method that enabled them to control a large, dynamic population of cultures and religious sects in India. Hindus don't remember this principle fondly, but we will employ a similar process with our breathing to effectively manage and control the complex energies that comprise our being.

Sectional breathing divides the lungs into three sections, which are worked with independently. The lower lungs control the root chakra, the sexual center, and the abdominal center; the mid-lung harmonizes the emotional center in the heart chakra; and the upper lung governs our expressive and perceptive sensitivities, namely the throat chakra and the command center between the eyebrows. When all three sections of the lungs are utilized, all six chakras are balanced and harmonized. Such complete breathing balances the energy and music of the body, guiding our streamlined energies toward the state of samadhi and enlightenment — the seventh chakra at the crown of the head.

For the following breathing exercises, you may sit in a meditation posture: cross-legged, between your heels, or on a chair.

Adhyam Pranayam: Reaching the Lower Lungs with Power Breathing

THE LOWER LUNGS can be used to tap into three basic levels of consciousness, associated with the first three chakras. First there is primal energy, associated with the base of the spine; next, the creative energy and passion linked to the genitals; and finally, organizational and motivational energy centered in the abdomen. These three spiritual powers — drive, creativity, and organization — are needed in our everyday working world as much as they are needed in the spiritual life.

The Method

IN POWER BREATHING, you will learn to breathe into the lowest regions of your lungs so that your abdomen is pushed outward. It is important to relax completely so that you can feel the action of your breath against your genitals and farther below, around the rectum, the base of the spine, and even in the lower back and hips. To experience your breath in these areas as you inhale gives a sense of security, vigor, and courage. When exhaling, gently contract your abdominal muscles and smoothly expel the air from your lower lungs. This is accomplished by coordinating the abdominal contraction with the regulation of breath in your throat. Obviously, you are employing the audible breath here, a technique you should use as much as possible. I also encourage you to exhale with your mouth open, making the audible sound "ah," and using the air in the lowest part of your lungs to create the sound. Then return to audible breathing with your mouth closed.

A Learning Tool

To better control your abdominal muscles, gently touch your fingertips to your navel. Maintain this light contact as you expand and contract your lower abdominal muscles. (Be careful not to push your abdomen with your fingertips during the contraction, and avoid obstructing the inflation of your abdominal area when expanding the lower lungs.) Once you get the hang of it, you can rest your hands on your knees and completely relax your body while you engage in this breathing technique. You can also place your palms on the sides of your hips to make sure the pressure is distributed all around your lower torso. When you coordinate your abdominal muscles with your breathing, you will become aware of a pressure building up in your pelvic area. This energy can be used sexually, or channeled farther up the spine to facilitate other ecstatic states.

Madhyam Pranayam: Heart-Space or Mid-Lung Breathing

In this exercise, you will isolate your breathing in your mid-lung area — around your solar plexus, which functions as the center point of your psycho-spiritual network and the seat of your emotional being. Cultures around the world regard this center as a place of balance and integrity because of its location close to the heart. Here our material and spiritual natures meet, and our masculine and feminine aspects find union.

Love, perception, and wisdom find their fulfillment when they come together in the heart. The heart is also the most obvious receptor and transmitter of energy among the chakras. It is easily "touched" when we are emotionally affected; it can be "gazed into" by the perceptive soul; and it can be "bared" to reveal the secrets of our innermost being to someone we trust. St. Benedict, the great father of Western monasticism (530 A.D.), invites his students to live the monastic rule by listening and inclining the ear of their hearts.[7] The word "courage," taken from the French, means "great heart." In so many ways, we can see that the totality of our human experience culminates in the heart. It is indeed the heart that best qualifies our essential nature: love.

The Method

EASE YOURSELF into your meditation position and become aware of your body as you breathe naturally. Focus your attention in the middle of your chest and observe the action of your breathing in that region. Take a slow, deep breath into your mid-chest and expand the space around your solar plexus, but avoid breathing into the top of your lungs.

A Learning Tool

TO GET A GOOD SENSE of how this is done, place your palms on the sides of your rib cage, midway between your hips and armpits. Press your thumbs against your back, and use the other fingers to hug the front of your rib cage. As you adjust your body to hold the position in comfort, you will naturally pick up on the action of your breathing in the mid-chest area, even if you do not breathe deeply. Send your breath into your palms, and you will notice your rib cage expanding outward when you breathe in, and returning to its original position when you breathe out. The effect is like playing an accordion.

Meditation

> **REGULATE THE FLOW** of breath in your throat and listen to its sound. You are also invited to use the audible sound "oh" (with your mouth open) on your exhalation. Later, close your mouth and use the audible breath to control airflow on the exhale. Rest whenever you need to, and resume the practice when you feel energized. Stay connected, and listen to what your body is telling you. Don't get too carried away by the emotional or spiritual states produced by your breathing practices;

keep your mind quiet and free from all deliberate activity. This doesn't mean that you won't have any thoughts at all, but stay connected with your breathing experience by constantly withdrawing from any involvement with your mental processes.

Adham pranayam: Upper-Lung or Brain-Stimulating Breathing

The region of the upper chest governs the throat center (associated with imagination, creativity, self-expression, and speech) and the wisdom center located between the eyebrows (associated with intuitive perception, cognitive knowledge, and the intellect). Upper-chest breathing stimulates the brain and all the creative, expressive, and perceptive powers of the higher Self.

You may have noticed that your upper chest becomes constricted when you are agitated or anxious, just as your abdomen tightens up when you are afraid. Learning to work with your breathing in your upper chest helps you channel your energies upward into your throat and head, then direct them toward the cosmic order and harmony of the universe known as rta — an expanded state that dissipates fear and anxiety. When done successfully, directing your energy into your head can generate clarity, receptivity, and deep insight. This realized energy can then be channeled downward to infuse your chakras with its special qualities. You will experience this when you combine all the sections of your lungs together in the great yogic breath.

The Method

Sit comfortably in your meditation posture and isolate your breathing in your upper chest, just below your collarbone, by keeping the middle and lower sections of your lungs relaxed. Next, breathe expansively into the upper region of your lungs so that your shoulder blades lift and your chest puffs up, and you look like a soldier on parade. You can also deliberately raise your shoulder blades to accommodate your breath in your upper chest and under your armpits. Once you understand the principle, allow your breathing to facilitate the movement.

A Learning Tool

YOU CAN FURTHER assist the process by placing your fingertips lightly on your upper chest or on your upper back, and allowing the contact of your fingertips with your body to guide you. You may also place your hands on your lower hips and observe the up-and-down movement of your shoulders as you breathe in and out. You will feel a rush of energy to your head as you do this.

Meditation

> Above all, do not forget to listen as you breathe audibly. Also, humming aloud on your exhalation will make your cranial area reverberate.

•

HAVING MASTERED these lung compartments independently, you will find it easy to perform the full-cycle breathing that employs all three of these regions in succession. If you have difficulty with full-cycle breathing, return to working with each section. Later, you can reapply the techniques to the complete breath known as the "great yogic breath," which we will explore in chapter fourteen.

> *When we study the science of breath, the first thing we notice is that breath is audible; it is a word in itself, for what we call "word" is only a more pronounced utterance of breath fashioned by the mouth and tongue. In the capacity of the mouth, breath becomes voice, and therefore the original condition of a word is breath. If we said, "First was the breath," it would be the same as saying, "In the beginning was the word."*
>
> **Hazrat Inayat Khanv**[8]

CHAPTER 14

SOUND

Sufi teacher Hazrat Inayat Khan once taught that the human voice is a barometer for the human soul. Its transparency reveals the soul's every condition. Joy, sorrow, anger, and pain — each has its own voice that comes through, despite the most skillful deception. Conversely, the Sufi path teaches that by affecting our voice, we can affect our soul, instilling in it the qualities we desire. In this chapter, we will learn the finer points of chanting practice through the sacred sound Om, a single mantric syllable that epitomizes the depth and power of Nada Brahman, the frequency that is God.

Why is the *Om* so important? First of all, the Om is tremendously sonorous; there appears to be no other mantra that can match its resonance in the human body. Regardless of your body's shape, this particular sound offers the maximum resonance possible. One objective of the sound yogi is to develop a resonant physical body through the regular use of sacred sound. Om is the single most important sound that can, by itself, configure the human body optimally for maximum resonance.

Secondly, this resonance is not static; the Om has a transparency that allows you to listen and perceive through its sound. Finally, the Om has an intrinsic ability to generate overtones. Overtones are the additional frequencies that occur over and above a tone; most tones are a mixture of the pure tone and these additional frequencies. Overtones are easily noticeable in acoustically resonant spaces, such as bathroom shower stalls, caves, or large cathedrals. Overtones are also produced in a resonant human body, and through the well-crafted tones of a trained vocalist. We naturally hear overtones when intoning the Om.

I recommend using a drone* while chanting the Om, or any mantra for that matter. Drones help generate undertones — frequencies that occur lower than the generated tone. These extended sounds are a foundation for healing; their sustained tones provide a sonic bed upon which to lie or an ocean in which to swim and explore our mantra practice. The standard drone is comprised of the root, fifth, and octave of the key you want to chant in. When undertones and overtones are produced together, as in the case of particularly long renditions of the *Om,* a quality of depth, connectedness, and healing issues forth from the mantra. "When the undertones are continuous, prolonged, and undisturbed, they function as a space for everything that healing music builds on."[1]

There are several other, more abstract, qualities of the mantra Om. First, the Om is universal; it leads us home to a place inside where we feel safe and secure, regardless of our cultural and religious affiliations. Next, the Om is self-contained, replete with its own fullness; it brings deep contentment to the user. Because it is so self-contained, the Om is also a self-propagating sound; the more you chant it, the more you are inspired to keep chanting it. Through its utter simplicity, the Om focuses our attention quickly, taking us inward and connecting us to our depth with the least encumbrance. Finally, the Om is mysterious; it awakens in us an immediate sense of the sacred that defies rational knowledge. This is paramount to yoga practice and mysticism from any cultural stream.

The Om is similar to its Christian counterpart, the "Amen." Both affirm the Divine presence, as they indisputably declare that the Divine is present, the Divine is all there is, and we are saying "yes" to its holy presence. Still, it doesn't take much experimentation to deduce that the Om is far more primal and suffused with resonance than the "Amen."

The Om is an ancient resonance that simulates the effect of a sonic womb. Physicist John Cramer of the University of Washington has

---

* A drone is a set of tones continually generated by a synthesizer, harmonium, sruti box, or stringed instrument like the tanpura. You may get yourself a drone CD from my Website (www.russillpaul.com).

created audio files simulating the sound of the "big bang," the birth of the universe.[2] He describes it thus: "The sound is rather like a large jet plane flying 100 feet above your house in the middle of the night."[3] If you listen to this sound develop, you will find it amazingly similar to the sound of a Tibetan monk overtoning* the sacred mantra Om.

Renowned yoga scholar Georg Feuerstein describes Om as follows:

> Om *is an experience rather than an arbitrary verbal label. It is a true symbol charged with numinous power. Experienceable in deep meditation, it is a sign of the omnipresence of* Ishvara *[the Divine] as manifest on the level of sound. . . . In other words, the human voice is employed to reproduce a "sound" which is continually "recited" by the universe itself— an idea, which in the Pythagorean School came to be known as the "harmony of the spheres." On the Indian side, it led to the development of the Yoga of Sound [Nada Yoga].*[4]

In chapter one, I mentioned the Swiss scientist Hans Jenny, who dedicated his life to the study of sound waves. Through a machine called the "tonoscope," he was able to visually represent patterns of sound. The tonoscope was constructed to make the human voice visible without any electronic apparatus as an intermediate link. This yielded a direct physical representation of the vowel, tone, or song of a human being, rendering a melody not only audible but visible.[5] Kay Gardner, in her book *Sounding the Inner Landscape,* tells us that the vowel "O" appears as a perfect circle in Jenny's tonoscope. More interestingly, the ancient Sanskrit mantra *Om,* when chanted into the tonoscope, shows not only the beginning "oh" sound, but also concentric diamonds and triangles within the circle formed by the harmonics during the *"mmmm"* at the end of the mantra. The image revealed is nearly identical to the *sri yantra*[6] (see illustration in chapter eight). The sri yantra is an ancient, complex mystical diagram of Hinduism, associated with the supreme goddess as matrix of the universe. A stunning connection, indeed!

The syllable Om represents the totality of Brahman. In Hinduism, the Om is also the Shabda Brahman, or "sonic absolute" that I discussed

* Tibetan overtone chanting is a technique in which vocal tones are manipulated by the lips, cheeks, throat, and tongue to produce a second note several octaves higher, which is superimposed on the first.

earlier, meaning that there is nothing higher than what it represents. Keep in mind that the audible Om produced through human vocal cords is only a simulation of a vast cosmic resonance that embraces the known universe. The audible Om represents *anahata nada,* an "unstruck" sounding — the spiritual presence of the unseen source of nature's cosmic intelligence, from which all the vibrations of the known universe emerge and into which they all disappear. Scientists call this "the field of indeterminate particles" — indeterminate because the particles appear and disappear without predictability. The only constant is the field itself; for the sound yogi, this is the field of consciousness — the fifth element of Sound Yoga (to be addressed in chapter sixteen).

Quantum physicists tell us that every measurable particle, however small, simultaneously exists as a wave of energy. Sound healer and tuning-fork expert John Beaulieu writes:

> *There is a similarity between cymatic pictures [the tonoscope pictures of Hans Jenny] and quantum particles. In both cases, that which appears to be a solid form is also a wave. They are both created and simultaneously organized by the principle of pulse. This is the great mystery with sound; there is no solidity! A form that appears solid is actually created by an underlying vibration.*[7]

DECONSTRUCTING THE MANTRA OM

The mantra Om is actually composed of four parts. Three of these parts are the distinct sounds "ah," "oh," and "mm" — the sounds you exhaled during the sectional breathing technique on page 169. The fourth is the silence that follows. The cosmic person known as *Purusha,* who is the universe, is said to be three-fourths in heaven and one-fourth on earth. You may recall that the same was said of Vak in chapter seven. The process of sounding the Om is broken down into these four parts, which form a progressive passageway between the manifest world of matter and energy and the unmanifest world of mind and Spirit. To understand this sonic passageway we shall look to the *Maitri Upanishad:*

> *There are two ways of contemplation of Brahman: in sound and in silence. By sound we go to silence. The sound of Brahman is Om.*

With Om we go to the End; the silence of Brahman. The End is immortality, union, and peace.

Even as a spider reaches the liberty of space by means of its own thread, the man [or woman] of contemplation by means of Om reaches freedom.[8]

This silence is not silence as we know it. It is not the absence of noise or external sound. It is, instead, that by which we are aware of sound; it is consciousness itself. All sound should lead to the experience of consciousness, which is a deep and complete awareness of the thing signified by the sound or word. Unfortunately, this doesn't happen very often. For the most part, we are content to communicate with labels, and to a large extent we are satisfied with a superficial awareness of what a word signifies. The powerful resonance and simplicity of the mantra Om reinstates consciousness in all our words, because Om truly represents — in sound and meaning — the totality of all that is and all that is not; it is both manifest universe and hidden mystery. You will find that your practice of this sound, coupled with a reverence for what it signifies, will lead to an enhanced experience in the way you communicate *any* sound, through any means.

Vacaspati, a famous Indian sage, explains a yogic technique of the interior apprehension of Nada Brahman through the mantra Om as follows:

Let the mind be concentrated upon the light shining in the lotus of the heart, which is located between the chest and abdomen. The eight petals of this lotus, which usually face downward, are reversed upward by the process of the expirative control of breath. In the middle thereof is the sphere of the sun, the place of waking consciousness, and it is called "A." Above that is the sphere of the moon, the place of dreaming consciousness, the "U." Above that is the sphere of fire, the place of dreamless sleep, the "M." Above that is the higher space, the sound of Brahman itself, the fourth state of ultra-consciousness.*[9]

THE OM AND CONSCIOUSNESS

EACH PART of the sacred Om corresponds to a particular state of consciousness: "A" corresponds to the waking state, "U" to the dream state,

* The Aum is the same as the Om. "Aum" is simply the way it's written, pronounced, and mystically interpreted. The practice on the accompanying audio tracks will help you understand how it sounds.

and "M" to the state of deep sleep. The silence that the Om resolves into is the fourth part of the mantra, which corresponds to the state of *turiya,* a field of spacious consciousness considered vital to the development of yogic power because it encompasses waking, dream, and deep sleep states in concurrent continuity.

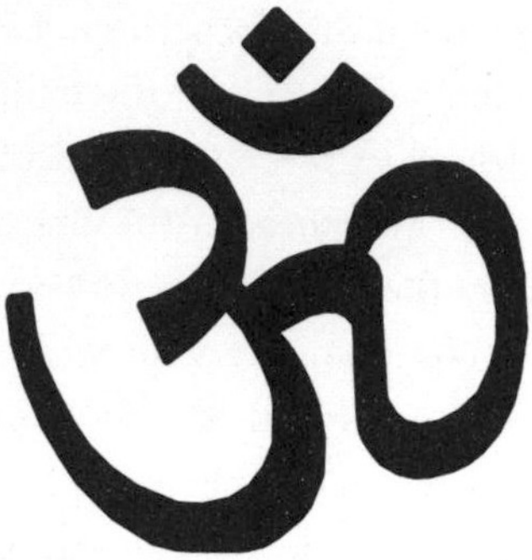

Even the visual symbol of the mantra Om is a mystical diagram that conveys this message of unified consciousness. The long, lower curve represents *jagrat,* the waking state and material existence. The extra length of this lower curve signifies the fact that the majority of human beings participate in this type of consciousness. The upper curve that picks up from the lower curve in the middle section of the letter represents deep and dreamless sleep, a state known as *susupti.* Between the two, a third coiled curve symbolizes the state of dreams, images from the unconscious and also intuitive thinking. Beyond these three states is the state of liberation, represented by the semicircle and the dot. The incompleteness of the semicircle signifies *maya,* the grand illusion and appearance of this world of forms, which beneath the surface is nothing but continually mobile waves of sound and energy. The dot represents illumination and turiya — the fourth state of consciousness, the silence of *Om.* Finite thinking cannot reach this point, which is separated from the flux of all existence.[10] It is the "still point of the soul" that Teilhard de Chardin spoke of — a place within us that no illusion can tarnish.

MAHAT YOGA PRANAYAMA: THE GREAT YOGIC BREATH

THE MOMENT the breathing stops, we know that the body of a living creature will die. Yet breathing is not continuous; there are pauses. Even the Divine, according to Tantric cosmology, requires breath cycles to continually recite the universe into being — and, like us, it pauses between breaths. This is known as *pralaya,* a process by which the energy and matter used to create forms recedes into the Divine abyss, then returns to the manifest world to renew the same forms or create new forms. Quantum physicists studying the behavior of subatomic particles corroborate this theory with their observations.

Meditating on the Om offers us the direct awareness that everything in the universe is held in existence by the Divine breath. This is why the great yogic breath is of utmost importance — for intoning not only the Om, but also other vowels. The production of sound in our body enables us to participate in the creative power of the Divine; by following the production of these tones, we can trace them back to their source in the quantum realm, and there discover the source of our own being.

Spiritual wholeness is achieved through the unified breath, which makes use of the various parts of the lung you have learned to control through the divide-and-rule method in the previous chapter. The great yogic breath is a complete way of breathing that involves every section of the lungs. It expels psychic toxins lodged in the body, clears blockages in the path of our energy flow, and invigorates the body's energy field with prana. In order to perform this great yogic breath, we must learn to coordinate the various parts of our lungs with the audible breath. To a musician, this is a bit like three-part harmony, except that the parts are successive, instead of simultaneous.

The purpose of this kind of breathing is to open every energy center, or chakra, located along the spinal cord and to clear any obstructions in the central pathway of energy that travels from the base of our spine to the top of our head. As we learned in chapter eight, a subtle body coexists with our physical body, with its own nervous system composed of psychic nerve channels called nadis. We achieve good health when the streams of our energy hum along these channels at optimal frequencies, particularly along the central susumna that travels up the spine.

The purpose of the great yogic breath *(Mahat Yoga Pranayama)* is to release the most primal form of the life force *(kundalini)* from the base of the spine, then raise it all the way to the top of the head. Like rivers on their way to the ocean, this primal energy gathers all the vibratory residues of unresolved past experiences on its upward journey, then merges with the sonic absolute, Shabda Brahman, at the top of the head. On its downward journey, this realized energy is allowed to impregnate every level of our being, right down to our roots. As our energy is allowed to travel freely up and down the spine, the circuitry of our entire nervous system is revitalized. This is the power of the great yogic breath.

The Method

Sit comfortably in your meditation position and relax. Observe your breath entering and leaving your body. Now take in a slow, deep breath and hold it for just an instant. When you start to exhale, retain maximum breath in your abdomen and release air from your upper chest first, causing the air from below, in the solar plexus region, to move into the upper chest and be forced out as well. Release air from your lower lungs only at the end of your exhalation by contracting your abdominal muscles. Regulate the flow of air in your throat, as described in the audible breath practice, so that you can control the entire process smoothly and achieve a progressive depletion of air pressure from the top down as you exhale. Employing the audible breath when you practice the great yogic breath will energize your body and lead you into profound states of meditation.

Hold the breath *outside* for a comfortable instant, then start to inhale. As you inhale, relax your abdominal muscles so that you can draw the air down into your gut, causing your belly to inflate. Continue to breathe, feeling this pressure rise into your solar plexus and upper chest until you are full of air. You will feel a lot of energy concentrated in your head.

Hold the breath *inside* for a comfortable moment, then start to exhale. Rest when you are tired or when you feel over-oxygenated. When you are rested, repeat the process.

Breath retention is important because these pauses between inhalation and exhalation are a form of sandhya, the merging of opposites that I mentioned earlier.

Some important tips: When first learning this practice, make sure that you don't contract your abdomen when you start to exhale — a normal tendency. You want to save this contraction for the end of the exhalation. Another common error is to contract the abdomen at the start of your inhalation. You must remember to relax the abdominal muscles you tensed at the end of your exhalation so that you can breathe into your lower lungs at the start of your inhalation. Otherwise, the abdominal tension will restrict your breathing into your mid-chest and upper chest.

The great yogic breath is essential to deriving the maximum energy from toning vowels — particularly when intoning the sacred syllable Om. This method, described with movements in chapter fifteen, is also helpful for singers, students of Indian music, and those who wish to lead Hindu devotional chanting.

CHANTING THE OM

There are many ways of chanting the Om, but the sound yogi takes into consideration the deep symbolism of the mantra and employs all the areas of the lungs and the muscle contractions of the great yogic breath while intoning the *Om*. This allows the fullness of the mantra's potency to be experienced while chanting.

It is common to purse one's lips to pronounce the mantra *Om*, especially because you see it written as "Om" in English. The Sanskrit character depicting the sound is written as "AUM," and it is pronounced accordingly, with "ah," "oh," and "mm" representing the three sonic parts of the mantra. When utilized in Sound Yoga, the mantra *Aum* begins with the vowel "ah" with the mouth wide open, jaws agape, taking care not to exaggerate the pronunciation of the opening vowel. You will notice that the fullest resonance of the "oh" sound ensues from this process.

Similarly, the middle vowel "oh" shouldn't be stretched out for too long unless you want to "tone" the sound, rather than chant it as a mantra (toning is prolonged vocalization of a vowel). Stretching out the vowel relaxes your jaw and facial muscles but doesn't bring about the specific spiritual power inherent in the mantra. It is important that the consonant "mm," which is the third part of the mantra, be vibrantly sounded so that it reverberates in the cranium. Through skillful contraction of the abdominal muscles, you should control this humming so that it smoothly tapers off into a silence of the body, mind, and heart. As you can see, the practice of the great yogic breath is necessary to derive the full benefit of this mantra. It shouldn't come as any surprise that the great yogic breath must accompany the great yogic sound.

The Method

Assume your meditation position and take a few moments to relax your face and shoulders. Keep your mind free from all deliberate activity; do not instigate, feed, or follow any of your thought processes.

1. Once you are mentally relaxed and acutely aware of your body, inhale deeply into your lower lungs. Remember to relax your abdominal muscles so that they can expand to accommodate your breath in the belly area. As your abdomen distends, allow your breath to fill your mid-chest, the sides of your rib cage, and finally the uppermost section of your lungs, just below your throat. Accomplish all this in a smooth, continuous inhalation.

2. Open your jaws wide and start to use the air in your upper chest to release the sound "ah," simultaneously retaining the maximum amount of air in your belly and mid-chest. The volume of air in your upper chest is small, so begin at a low pitch and keep your opening vowel short.

3. Quickly launch the "ah" into an "oh" on a slightly raised pitch by using the air from your mid-chest. Try to get the sound to resonate in your upper body, and develop the sound so that it builds slightly in volume; it will appear to rise up from your belly into your chest. You will need to coordinate all this with your abdominal muscles in a way that continues to retain breath in the lower lungs, which must be saved for the "mm" that concludes the mantra.

4. As you develop the "oh" sound, begin to close your mouth; this naturally changes the vowel into the consonant "mm." Resolve the "mm" by gradually contracting your abdominal muscles and using only a minimum amount of air. The "mm" resonates strongly in the cranium. Conclude the sound smoothly, gradually diminishing its intensity and volume with a pleasant transition into silence. Your awareness will naturally be drawn to your forehead, where you will notice a slight throbbing, particularly when you run out of

breath. This is normal, as the process awakens the third eye of intuitive perception, the eye of Shiva.

5. Pause for a brief moment, holding your breath outside. When you inhale, allow your breath to pass through the throbbing sensation in your forehead. Always send your breath down to your lower lungs first to inflate those abdominal muscles that have been drawn in, then breathe into your mid-lungs, and finally, top off your lungs by allowing air into the uppermost section, just below your throat. Get ready for your second Om.

You may perform three Om mantras in this manner, rest briefly, then do two more sets of three Om mantras. That's a total of nine Om mantras in three sets.

The bow is the sacred Om, the arrow is our own soul.
Brahman is the mark of the arrow, the aim of the soul.
Even as an arrow becomes one with its mark,
let the watchful soul be one in him [the Divine].

Mundaka Upanishad[11]

CHAPTER 15

MOVEMENT

All sound generates the movement of energy. Mantras, in particular, can create powerful surges of energy flow that seek expression in movement. Conversely, all movement configures, releases, and distributes energy, but some movements do so better than others. In dance, Hatha Yoga, and Tai Chi, energy is configured in a harmonious pattern; good movement feels like good music, and vice versa. It is also important to understand the dynamics of motion inherent in sound, which we will explore in this chapter.

As we have seen in chapters seven through ten, movement within the streams of traditional Sound Yoga is extremely varied. In the Vedic Shabda tradition, movement is expressed through a rich assortment of delicate ritual gestures and actions performed in a precise manner; failure to do so destroys the purity and potency of the ritual. One such traditional set of gestures, *Sandhya Upaasana,* is described in appendix one. In the Tantric tradition, movement is represented through internal muscle contraction, complex breathing techniques, and the subtle posturing of the hands called "mudras." I have addressed some of these gestures on the accompanying audio tracks as well as in appendix two. Wild dancing and cathartic movements are also associated with the awakening of energy in certain Tantric ceremonies and in temples dedicated to the goddess, particularly in South India. In the Bhakti tradition, we find the informal movement of gentle body swaying, snapping of fingers, and dancing with ecstatic abandon. As is the case with devotional mantras, the devotional movements of the Bhakti tradition are unrestricted and free from the precise rules of Vedic and Tantric practice.

POETRY IN MOTION

MOVEMENT IN YOGA is well represented through Hatha Yoga practice; it is precisely for this reason that Hatha Yoga complements the Yoga of Sound so well. Hatha Yoga has aptly been described as "poetry in motion." While mantras are traditionally used in a number of the meditation postures, many readers will be surprised that, for the most part, mantras are not combined with many of the flowing postures, which require much care and concentration. But some Hatha Yoga schools, such as Swami Sivananda's Integral Yoga, pair twelve Vedic mantras with the sun salutation, a series of twelve interconnected postures. These twelve movements may also be used with the six Tantric bijas *hraam, hreem, hroom, hraim, hroum,* and *hrah,* which are chanted twice in that order to complete the entire sequence. Sometimes Tantric and Vedic mantras are combined in a devotional format during the sun salutation. An example is *Om Hreem Ra-va-ye Namaha.* See appendix two for a full list.

There is still much room for the incorporation of motion in Sound Yoga, especially pairing deliberate, harmonious movements with mantras. In my experience, many Western spiritual seekers yearn for such movement; they are not accustomed to sitting for long periods of time and may want more than an interior process and prescribed gestures, at least when newly exploring yoga.

You may wonder where Indian dance, with its elaborate vocabulary of expression and movement, fits into yoga. Dance, known as *natya,* is considered to be an aspect of music in the Hindu tradition because it expresses line, color, proportion, movement, rhythm, and harmony — all musical principles. Yet neither Indian classical dance nor Indian classical music is appropriate for the general practitioner of Sound Yoga because of their focus on performance and the high standards of artistic refinement that accompany the training process. Such demands may actually stand in the way of an interior apprehension. The emphasis on technique and technical rigor often overpower the openness necessary for a beginning Sound Yoga practice. It is perhaps best to view Indian classical music and Indian dance as advanced practices of Sound Yoga and Hatha Yoga.

So how do we come up with a working vocabulary of motion for the beginner in Sound Yoga? Because movement is so therapeutic, I believe it is extremely important that various forms of movement, even freestyle motion, be incorporated into Sound Yoga practice. A certain amount of creative freedom will certainly make our explorations of Sound Yoga more personal and more exciting. But what we are looking for is deliberate, coordinated movement that works with sound and mantra.

Over the past twenty years of study and developing a personal practice, I have found a number of movements conducive to the practice of sacred sound. Many of these movements and gestures are authentic to India, inspired by religious ceremonies or folk dancing in the temples, some of which I will share with you in this chapter. Others are adapted Sufi practices, such as the *Zikr* and *Sama,* which I will describe. Some movements are derived from Tai Chi and Chi Gong, such as the motions of vowels that I describe in this chapter and on the accompanying audio tracks. We won't create an eclectic hodgepodge of jazz ballet or aboriginal tribe movements, however. In all instances, I have tried to maintain an atmosphere of consciousness authentic to the Hindu tradition, using only those movements that enhance the power of the sounds.

ZIKR AND SAMA: CHANTING AND MOTION IN SUFISM

IT WAS THE SUFIS, Islam's underground mystical movement, who truly incorporated a vast vocabulary of movements and gestures into their sonic meditations. Not surprisingly, Sufism was very much in dialogue with Hinduism and its esoteric yogic practices, but it developed its own sacred movements and mystical tradition of sound along parallel, yet separate, lines. Zikr, the remembrance of God, represents the mantra tradition within Sufism. Zikr is often combined with Sama, the Sufi's mystical dance-like movements, usually performed with raga-like music. The circular motion of whirling dervishes is a key Sama practice, which was institutionalized by the Mevlevi order. Rumi, the founder of the Mevlevi and the most famous advocate of Sama, described the dance as "movement induced by the vision of the beloved, who himself may dance on the screen of the lover's heart in the hour of ecstasy."[1]

Legend has it that Rumi had been missing his beloved friend, Shamsuddin of Tibriz, a vagabond spiritual alchemist and Divine manifestation of the cosmic teacher. Shams was a great awakener of love in Rumi's life, but jealous students had forced Shams to leave the premises of Rumi's school of sacred learning. Distraught with grief, Rumi was in the marketplace one day when he heard Shams call his name. Taken by surprise, but unsure if it was indeed Shams calling out to him, Rumi cupped an ear with one hand in order to hear better and held out the other hand in longing expectation. The sound changed direction, and Rumi's body turned. He heard his name called out repeatedly, and the source constantly moved, tracing a circle around the marketplace. As Rumi's body responded to each call, it naturally began to spin ecstatically.

There are as many forms of Zikr as there are Tariqats (Sufi Orders) and Shaykhs (leaders) within these orders. Usually a Zikr is held in a space that is empty except for a prayer carpet on the floor. Sometimes there is a special rug or sheepskin for the leader. In traditional settings, the men are seated apart from the women. Generally, following the leader, the group chants or recites evocative words, the names of God in Arabic, and musical prayers similar to Hindu devotional chanting. Movements may accompany the words. The whirling often associated with the dervish ceremony is done only in special situations.[2]

The use of mantric phrases in some Sufi communities is performed by sitting on the heels (like vajrasana), their elbows close to each other, and making simultaneous light movements of the head and body. In other settings, the movement consists of balancing oneself, swaying gently from right to left and left to right, or inclining the body methodically forward and backward.[3] In yet other situations, the Zikr movement would be to plunge the head first toward one knee and then toward the other, the intention being to dive deep into the heart and back out again. It could be said that the bobbing motion that Jews perform in prayer at the wailing wall in Jerusalem is a form of Zikr.[4]

In some Sufi Orders, such as the *Kadirees* and the *Rufa'ees,* the exercises are performed by first holding hands in a circle, then putting the right foot forward to rotate the body with hands free, and increasing the strength of the movement by using the foot as an accelerator. Known as the *Devr,* which may be translated as "dance" or "rotation," this practice closely parallels Hindu circumambulation, a popular form of meditative motion done while chanting mantras. The duration of these Sufi dances is not fixed; each person is free to leave when he or she pleases. However, the dancers make it a point to remain in session as long as possible. The strongest, most robust, and most enthusiastic strive to persevere longer than the others; they take off their turbans, form a second circle within the other, entwine their arms within those of their brethren, lean their shoulders against each other, gradually raise their voices, and, without ceasing, repeat "Ya Allah!" (Oh, God) or "Ya Hu" (Oh, He), increasing the movement of their bodies, and not stopping until their strength is exhausted.[5] This is how Sound Yoga should be practiced: by holding nothing back and chanting until all karma has been burned up in the flames of devotion.

The Dances of Universal Peace, a chant and movement meditation developed by the American Sufi Murshid Samuel Lewis, combine Zikr with communal motions. This type of Zikr is widely practiced in the West among American Sufis; Hindu mantras such as *Shree Ram Jai Ram* are often utilized.

Tai Chi and Chi Gong are also powerful representations of sound and energy expressed in motion. What is wonderful about Tai Chi, Chi Gong, and Sufi dancing is that these movements are not really external. Rather, they facilitate interiority and work efficiently with internal energy.

A Simple Zikr and Sama Practice

The following Zikr and Sama is an adaptation of the whirling motion of Sufi dervishes. This motion is much slower, allowing us to touch our deep center and respond to the call of the Beloved in our heart. I first learned the motion in a workshop session with Pir Vilayat Khan, the son of Hazrat Inayat Khan; the palm-gazing technique I devised from inspiration. Sufis note that turning clockwise directs our energy into the heart; spinning or turning counterclockwise allows our energy to flow outward into the world. The practice of Zikr is used to "remember" the Beloved and awaken to the Divine presence in the heart. Any devotional mantra may be employed for this practice. You may rotate your body in silence, while you chant, or with evocative music or chanting in the background.

The Method

1. Place your left palm over your heart and connect with the source of love in your body. Hold your right palm up like a mirror and gaze deeply into it, as though you were gazing deeply into your soul. Sense the Divine presence all around you by becoming aware of the vibratory presence of sacred energy in the cellular structures of your body.

   Sufi mystic Ibn Al Arabi once wrote, "The eye through which you see God is the same eye through which God sees you." Hindus call this *darshan,* which is the grace of simultaneously seeing and being seen by the Divine. It is darshan that inspires a Hindu to worship in a temple, meet a holy person, or travel to a sacred place. Let this be your experience as you gaze into your palm.

2. Begin to move your right palm to the right, and trace a slow, continuous circle around your body. The rest of your body will naturally follow the palm, allowing the wisdom of your body to take over. Remember the decapitated skulls around Kali's neck? All too often, our experiences of prayer are confined to our head; this is a way to pray with our body.

   There is an amazing story from the tradition of Christian Hermeticism,* a Gnostic school within Christianity. As Dionysus was walking near a place called Marmion, he suddenly realized that his head had been severed from his body. So he turned around, walked back, picked up his head, and, placing it under his arm, continued on his journey.[6] This

* Hermeticism is an esoteric Gnostic tradition dating back to the third century A.D. in the Egyptian desert, where many hermits, including Christian monks, lived. A mythic figure known as Hermes Trismegistus is credited with ancient texts known as the *Corpus Hermeticum,* a Hellenistic fusion of the Greek god Hermes and the Egyptian god Thoth. See Phillip J. Brown's article, "Hermeticism" at http://www.belinus.co.uk/mythology/Hermeticism.htm.

insightful story describes that moment of mystical grace when the Divine intervenes in our lives and shows us that we must surrender our cerebral center to our rhythmic center, permitting the body to lead the mind. Allow this intervention to guide your body prayer.

3. Your motion should be slow, continuous, and mindful. Alternatively, you may turn freely, sometimes opening both arms lovingly so that the Divine presence can embrace your soul or vice versa. If you become dizzy, you may anchor your left heel on the floor and swivel around it.

4. You can use any mantra for this practice, but to learn the method I suggest the Vedic mantra *Om Ee-shaa Vaa-syam Idham*. This is the first line of the *Eesha Upanishad,* which Gandhi considered a profound summary of all Hindu experience. The word *Eesha* means "all-powerful One," and its wind-like, fluid sound has a pervasive quality that works well with the next word, *Vaa-syam,* which means "to dwell, be worn as clothing, be perfumed by, or pervade by." *Idham* means "all this, here, this body, this world, this place." The chant therefore means: "All this is pervaded by the perfume of the Divine presence." Gandhi liked to say, "If Christians truly want to convert others, they must preach by their perfume, not by their words." This means giving off good vibes wherever we go, speaking by our presence — a wonderful way of bearing witness to our spiritual truths.

   Take in a slow, deep breath and sing out *Om Ee-shaa Vaa-syam Idham,* all in a single breath. Take in another slow breath and repeat the chant. Keep drawing in a slow, deep breath between each sounding of the mantra as you turn.

5. After a while, whisper the mantra on your breath, still turning. Later, intone the mantra in your mind as you turn. Eventually, come to a standstill and center yourself in your heart. Maintain an interior silence, and enjoy the powerful sense of union you feel with the Beloved.

Other mantras you can use with this practice are:

Om Namah Shivaaya ("I worship the dance of creation")
Om Namah Christaaya ("I worship the presence of Christ")
Om Namah Durgaaya ("I worship that fierce, feminine light that burns away all impurity")

CIRCUMAMBULATION

Circumambulation — walking around a shrine or sacred site as part of a ritual — is one of Hinduism's most common movement meditations. A story often associated with this practice describes Ganesh and Murugan, the two sons of Shiva and Parvati, vying for a sacred gift. It was decreed that whoever went around the cosmos three times and returned first would receive the gift. Murugan flew off on his vehicle, the peacock. Ganesh, a spiritual power associated with knowledge and learning, knew that his vehicle, the mouse, was no match for Murugan's peacock. So Ganesh devised an ingenious method of claiming the gift: he reverently circled his parents three times. In Tantric cosmology, Shiva and Shakti together make up the entire universe, so Ganesh was essentially circling the cosmos. He won the sacred gift.

Circumambulation in a temple, in front of a shrine, or around a holy tree is always done a minimum of three times to signify that all levels of consciousness are affected. Equally common is standing in one place and turning around one's own central axis, a familiar sight on Indian streets throughout the day. A common utterance during circumambulation is one's core mantra, or the mantra of the deity dwelling in the shrine where one is worshipping. Popular mantras while circumambulating include *Shiva Shiva; Raam Raam;* and *Om Shakti.*

The power of circumambulation is protection. Another function is purification, as in Islam, in which circling the Haaj restores one's relationship with the Divine. Hindus will often say, "May I become free from all past transgressions," as they circumambulate. In Hinduism, circumambulation is known as *pradakshina,* a Sanskrit word meaning "moving rightward, or clockwise." The intention is to shift the mind from worldly concerns to an awareness of the Divine, much like the Zikr's "remembrance." Clockwise movement is considered to raise awareness from the lower chakras upward, while the reverse moves awareness downward into the lower chakras. Clockwise motion is preferred in Hinduism.

When circumambulating, it is popular to join the palms all the way above the head while turning. This gesture is reserved for the holy of holies, and used only in the presence of the most high. By contrast, the "namaste" greeting, used to honor fellow human beings, is performed by joining the palms at the heart, a gesture known as *anjali mudra*. When placed at the forehead, this mudra establishes a sacred connection between the mind and the object of one's devotion. This position is often used to venerate spiritual teachers.

HOPPING, STOMPING, SWAYING, AND GYRATING

GENTLE SWAYING is a wonderful motion to use while chanting. In fact, it is natural and spontaneous when singing kirtans. Try a swaying motion as you chant the mantra *Shree Raama Jai Raama Jai Jai Raamo.*

Gyrating — rotating your torso or hips in small and large circles — is particularly effective when using Shakti mantras, as it causes energy to swirl with the objective of removing toxicity from our system. You can do this by sitting and rotating your torso 360 degrees in repeated circles, or by standing and rotating your hips in the same manner.

A powerful image associated with this motion is the churning of the cosmic ocean by the *Devas* (beings of the sky, associated with light) and *Asuras* (forces of the earth, fertility powers associated with the dark). The ocean symbolizes the unconscious. A story in the Hindu *Puranas* describes how these two groups, both parts of ourselves that desire immortality, need to work together in order to produce transformation. When we bring together our earthiness (the incarnate aspect of our being) with the subtle spiritual aspect of our being, Divine nectar is produced through this yoga. Reciting a mantra while you gyrate is thus a means of churning our own cosmic ocean; the mingling energies of our physical and mental dimensions awaken our immortality. Try chanting the mantra *Om Namah Shivaa-ya, Shivaa-ya Namah Om* — a mantra palindrome — while you gyrate.

Stomping the feet, usually in rhythm, symbolizes the destruction of ignorance. One instance of this metaphor is found in Shiva's classic posture as *Nataraja,* the Lord of the Dance, in which he has one foot on a dwarf, who represents ignorance. Another is that of Kali poised with one foot above a reclining, submissive Shiva, symbolizing the ultimate transformation of libido in Tantric practice. Try chanting the mantra *Om Shakti Om Shakti Om Shakti Om* as you stomp your feet in rhythm.

One variation of hopping, in the Tantric style, is to spread your feet apart and stretch out both hands fully on each side, palms facing downward. Next, turn to the right and hop in that direction, lifting both feet off the ground each time. Reverse the process. Use the mantra *Aadhi Shakti, Aadhi Shakti, Aadhi Shakti Om; or Mahaa Shakti, Mahaa Shakti, Mahaa Shakti Om* as you hop. Tantric devotees move this way when infused with the energy of the goddess.

Another variation is performed by hopping from one foot to another. This is an ecstatic motion employed by Bhaktas as well as Tantrics to induce trance states. The Hare Krishnas often use this technique. Try chanting the maha mantra *Ha-re Raa-ma, Ha-re Raa-ma, Raa-ma, Raa-ma, Ha-re, Ha-re; Ha-re Krish-na, Ha-re Krish-na, Krish-na Krish-na, Ha-re, Ha-re* as you hop from one foot to the other in rhythm with the chant. Start slowly, build up speed, and then slowly resolve to a standstill.

MOTION OF VOWELS: THE DIRECTIONALITY OF SOUND

As much as we want to move our bodies when we employ sacred sound, it is equally important to learn to perceive the movement that is inherent "within" sound. All sound has direction encoded within its shade of vowel, pitch, and timbre. Vowels, in the ancient Vedic tradition, were associated with *Indra.* One of the principal deities of the early Vedic world, Indra is the god of thunder and the first deity to be formally associated with the power of sacred sound.

The vowel sounds — O, A, E, and U — have great transparency, as evident from "ooh" (as in "woo"), expressing delight; "aah," declaring wonder; "eek," a nervous shriek; and "oh," registering surprise or curiosity. Notice, too, that each of these expressions carries with it a distinctive pitch: "ooh" and "oh" are usually low, "aah" is moderate, while "eek" is invariably high-pitched.

Pitch, as we know, has directionality. Physics explains low tones as slower-moving sound waves that act upon the denser parts of the body;

the reason we start moving our tailbone the moment we enter a nightclub or discotheque is because the low boom of a bass guitar or the thump of a bass drum reverberates in our depths. High pitches are rapid frequencies that affect the subtle consistencies of our being, such as our brain. A "hot" solo from a violin goes quickly to our head. This is why composers often have solo instruments like the violin or viola play over the orchestra, since they can literally cut through the sound from the other instruments. Similarly, we tend to speak in a higher pitch when we are excited or trying to cut through someone's thoughts and get their attention. Conversely, we speak in a lower pitch after having awakened from a good night's sleep; we are relaxed, and our consciousness resides in a deep place.

In the Tibetan Tantric tradition of yoga, the mantras *hoom* and *hrih,* (pronounced "hree"), which contain the vowels U and E, are considered complementary to each other in their energetic direction. *Hrih* is said to have the nature of flame — a shooting-upward quality that moves rapidly toward the head and skyward.

Complementing the mantra *hrih* is the mantra *hoom,* which has a descending, downward motion. Even the visual representation of this sound in English, "U," depicts a downward plunge.

The vowel O has an inclusive, circular motion that seems to gather all things into itself — a powerful feminine quality. The mantra *Om* is composed using this vowel, and it is no coincidence that it is visually represented as a circle. The oscilloscope, a modern instrument used to "see" sound, displays the shape of the vowel O as a circular image. The sound "O" is like the womb from which all things come forth, and the "ocean," into which all sounds ultimately merge.

The vowel A ("ah") is definitely a heart sound, found in words such as "heart" and "art." The sound "ah" has a horizontal, outgoing, extroverted quality, which I like to think of as moving across the surface of the earth to embrace all creatures.

Finally, the vowel I, which combines the vowels A and E, appears to be a solitary, stationary sound; it is centered in the self and points to the self. I also rhymes with words such as "eye," an organ that sees things as separate from one another; "ice," a frozen substance; and "island," meaning "that which is isolated." On a positive note, the holy syllable

Aim, pronounced like the English contraction "I'm," is associated with *Saraswati,* the goddess of wisdom and learning; it is known as the "guru-bija," or the seed-syllable of the teacher. Let us, therefore, view this vowel as a sound that centers us in the deep self, the true self, the authentic self within. The meaning of the word "Saraswati" is "she who flows." Originally the name of one of the holiest rivers in the Vedic world, Saraswati was also the name given to Brahma's consort. Brahma is the creator principle in the Hindu Trinity, and Saraswati is his "shakti," his force. The bija mantra *Aim* and its vowel I can be used to visualize all streams of energy flowing in and out of the deep self.

In the following exercise, we will take the key components of Sound Yoga that we have addressed thus far — posture, breath, and sound — and work them into movements. Unless otherwise instructed, prevent your hands and fingertips from touching for all these exercises. Keeping your hands apart allows for a certain charge of energy to develop between your palms.

Circle of Power

1. FEELING THE SOUND: Stand with your feet apart, knees slightly bent, and palms at your heart, separated but facing each other; your fingers are pointing upward. This is your base position. First, empty your lungs completely — top first, bottom last. Now fill your lungs, section by section, starting with the lower lungs. Choose a comfortable tone for expressing the vowel "oh." As you tone the vowel on exhalation, first use air from the upper portion of your lungs, then the mid-chest, and finally the abdomen. After you have produced the tone, draw your breath in slowly and audibly through both nostrils. Observe how the energy generated by the tone moves around in your body. To obtain the full effects of this practice, use your body as a sounding board or resonating chamber instead of projecting your voice into the room.
2. GAINING CONTROL: Produce the "oh" softly at first by using the air from your upper chest. Next, move rapidly into

developing the sound in volume and resonance by using the air from your mid-chest; the abdominal area should retain its air. The moment you have used the air from your mid-chest, your abdominal muscles will begin to contract; use this contraction as your cue to resolve the tone smoothly with air from your lower lungs, allowing the sound to taper off into silence. With practice, you will be able to produce a steady, uninterrupted tone that builds and resolves smoothly.

You are initiating, developing, and resolving the tone into silence. This is participation in the Divine act of creation, following the process to its source in the Absolute Sound.

3. ENHANCING THE TONE WITH MOVEMENT: The sound "oh" has a circular movement. As you tone the sound, imagine it as a spherical ball of energy that is exploding gently within your being and unfolding multidimensionally through you. Position your hands at your forehead in a pyramid shape, with your fingertips gently touching. Begin to trace the shape of this spherical sound with your palms as you intone the vowel, each hand tracing a semicircle down either side of your body and resolving into a complete circle that culminates at the base of your spine. Visualize your body as the galaxy, with your breath spiraling around your heart, the sun. When inhaling, direct the movement of energy up your spine, following the ascent of your breath with your palms until they return to your forehead in the pyramid shape you began with. Repeat the vowel "oh" several times until you feel the experience come together for you. This exercise helps unify a fragmented personality or a distracted mind.

Igniting the Flame

1. FEELING THE SOUND: Stand with your feet apart, knees slightly bent, hands positioned as though you were holding a large bowl at chest height, palms facing upward, elbows comfortably close but not pressing against the body. This

time, use the vowel-sound "ee," and choose a high tone to express it. Observe the direction of the sound as it moves in your body.

2. GAINING CONTROL: Gain control as you did with the previous vowel, using air from the various sections of your lungs to initiate, develop, and resolve the intensity of the tone. Wasn't it worth working on that sectional breathing?
3. ENHANCING THE TONE WITH MOVEMENT: Position your hands and body as described in "Feeling the Sound." Inhale, filling your lungs with air from the bottom upward. As you tone the high-pitched "ee," slowly raise your palms upward, as though they were magnetically attracted to the sky. When you reach the level of your face, branch off your hands on either side with palms leading, as though a fountain were sprouting from the top of your head. As you allow your hands to descend on either side of your body, sink down by bending your knees.
4. As you inhale, straighten your knees and allow your palms to ascend alongside the spine, following your breath toward your chest. When your lungs are filled, you will be ready to repeat the sound and movement.

Notice how the vowel seems to push through the crown of your head as it seeks release in the space above your head. Visualize your energy breaking through your head and stimulating your brain cells. This exercise helps charge your brain with creative energy.

Expanding Your Heart

1. FEELING THE SOUND: Stand with your feet apart, palms positioned in front of your body, as though you were protecting your breasts, with your elbows sticking out to either side. The fingertips of both hands should be pointing at each other, your thumbs bent downward, and the centers of your

palms aligned with your nipples. Tone the vowel-sound "ah" and feel its motion in your body.

2. GAINING CONTROL: Work on initiating, developing, and resolving the tone smoothly, as before.

3. ENHANCING THE TONE WITH MOVEMENT: Position your hands and body as described in "Feeling the Sound." Take in a slow, deep breath and fill your lungs from the bottom upward. You should experience your palms and elbows rising slightly as the energy fills your lungs. When you begin to tone the sound "ah," start to move your palms away from your body; spread your fingers so that they become web-like and keep moving your arms outward until you are stretched out like Christ on the cross. As you tone the sound, allow your energy to bless all living creatures over the face of the earth. When inhaling, slowly draw your palms back to where they were when you started, matching your breathing with the motion of your hands. Repeat the exercise a few times. This is a great way to release anger, emotional pain, and tension.

Descending into the Depths

1. FEELING THE SOUND: Stand relaxed with your knees slightly bent. Position your palms at your chest, facing downward, with your elbows bent and out to the sides. Choose a low pitch — as low as possible without being too soft or lacking energy. Bend your head slightly downward with your chin pressing toward your collarbone, but keep your chest up; this will help you produce a clear, stable tone using the vowel U, as in the word "who" but without the aspiration. Make sure it isn't an "oh." Notice the direction of the sound moving in your body, and make sure that your spine stays relaxed and erect.

2. GAINING CONTROL: Follow the same process you did with the other vowels, ensuring that your tone is not wobbly. A gradual contraction of your abdominal muscles

will help push the sound deep into your pelvic area and toward the base of your spine.

3. ENHANCING THE TONE WITH MOVEMENT: Stand with your hands and body positioned as described in "Feeling the Sound." As you inhale, slowly raise your arms straight upward, as though you were gathering an armload of energy. When your palms meet above your head, push straight downward along your body as you tone the vowel U. Midway through your descent (around your heart-space), start to bend your knees; keep your spine straight, being mindful not to lean forward.

   As you sound this vowel, imagine your energy plunging into the depths of your consciousness and settling deep, deep down. You will find a center in the very pit of your being where such stability and strength feel natural. Use your palms to follow the movement of your energy and intention downward. When you have completed the tone, slowly straighten your knees and raise your arms outward on either side, as though you were gathering another armload of energy to channel through your being a second time. Repeat the exercise. Use this practice when you feel frazzled, insecure, or out of your depth, and it will help you to quickly regain your balance.

Centering

For the last vowel, "I" (pronounced "eye"), stand with your feet together and palms joined at your heart in the namaste position. Inhale through your nostrils, drawing your breath into your solar plexus, then exhale through your open mouth while whispering the sound "I" softly into your heart-space to invoke a deep sense of self — deeper than all thoughts and images, deeper even than dreams.

Dancing the Vowels

In this exercise, you will combine all five vowels and their movements to invoke a multidimensional energetic space through sound.

You may also combine the vowels with consonants, which add thrust to the vowels, transforming them into the bija mantras *Om, Hrih, Ma, Hoom,* and *Aim*. These jewel-like sounds are very powerful.

A brief note for the musically inclined: Choose a comfortable octave to work with, and try this exercise using the tonic for the "oh," or *Om;* the higher octave for "ee," or *hrih;* the middle fifth for "ah," or *ma;* and the lower, deep fifth for "ooh," or *hoom*. The "I," or *aim,* is expressed without pitch. For example: middle C, G, the octave C, and then the G below middle C will be the notes for the key of C. The fifths create stability and balance, while the tonic and octave offer unity and a sense of completeness. The first four sonic motions performed together will move your energy through all the chakras. I compare this to St. Paul's eloquent description of knowing the height, length, breadth, and depth of Divine love. The fifth vowel and mantra will center you.

The Method

1. Start with your feet apart and knees slightly bent. With your palms facing downward, breathe in slowly and deeply while raising your palms toward your head. Begin to tone the *Om* as you exhale while tracing the sound and shape of the mantra in a circular fashion, as though caressing a sphere. Your palms meet at the genital area, facing upward. Keep your spine straight, but bend your knees a bit more toward the latter half of your exhalation so that the space between your thighs opens up as you conclude the sound.
2. With bent knees and palms joined below the abdomen (facing upward), take a slow, deep breath, directing the air into the lowest regions of your lungs. Match the upward flow of breath with your palms, moving them straight upward as you continue breathing, now into your solar plexus. When your palms arrive at your chest and your upper lungs are filled with air, begin a high-pitched *hrih* as you exhale and straighten your knees. Use the aspiration to propel energy into your head, which you will follow with your palms,

pushing upward and branching off at the top of your head to create a fountain-like effect.

3. As you inhale, spread your arms wide apart and let them descend slowly on either side of your body, eventually bringing your hands together at your heart, palms facing your chest.
4. Tone the mantra *ma* on your exhalation, palms moving outward and fingers stretching apart until both arms are stretched out on either side.
5. Take in a slow breath as you gather an armload of energy, and tone the mantra *hoom* with palms facing downward and pushing toward the genitals. Bend your knees halfway through your exhalation and keep your spine straight.
6. Breathe in slowly, bringing your feet together, raising your palms, and joining them at your heart. Exhale through your mouth while you softly whisper the mantra *aim*. Stand still for a few moments and allow the effects of your practice to be distributed throughout your body as you breathe normally.

VARIATIONS:

- Repeat this five-step process two more times, for a set of three complete cycles.
- Perform one set of three cycles with the vowels, and one set of three with the bija mantras.
- Perform one set of three cycles with the vowels, a second set of three cycles with the bija mantras, and a third set of three cycles whispering the vowels on your breath without tones.

SOME TIPS: For best results, resolve each sound smoothly. Coordinate your breathing with the sounds you are producing, synchronizing breath and sound with your body movements. The exercise becomes even more powerful when the great yogic breath and the audible breath are employed, opening a multidimensional energetic space through sound.

FREEDOM OF EXPRESSION, GROUNDED IN DEPTH

ALL TOO OFTEN, yoga practice is very formal, and much of Western spirituality is overly educated and too much in the head. Sometimes this center of reference must be severed, and what better way to do this than through mantra combined with movement? On many occasions, I encourage my students to let their bodies do as they please for a period of time, usually at the climax of the chanting. I always begin my "body prayers" with traditional movements, either Hindu or Sufi, develop the practice into wild abandon, then return to a deep stillness and silence. I recommend that you keep this cycle in mind when you design your own body prayers with mantras. As you experiment with motions to complement mantric utterances, also keep in mind the sacredness of these mantras.

CHAPTER 16

CONSCIOUSNESS

Each of the four elements previously described in this section — posture, breath, sound, and movement — embodies a specific stream of Sound Yoga. Posture embodies shabda, the word; breath embodies shakti, energy; movement embodies bhava, or devotion; and, of course, sound embodies nada, the flowing current of sound itself. The fifth element of Sound Yoga — consciousness — is the natural by-product of all of these elements and streams. When all the elements and streams work together seamlessly as an integrated practice, the experience of pure consciousness is unveiled. This is samadhi, the ultimate goal of yoga and of all spiritual endeavors.

We began chapter one with the idea that our species is suffering from an imbalance. "Human beings, with their disproportionate emphasis on seeing, have brought on the excess of rationality, of analysis and abstraction, whose breakdown we are now witnessing," claims musicologist and sonic scholar Joachim-Ernst Berendt.[1] Berendt further explains that the emerging "new consciousness," or "new thought" movement, which has been at the forefront of many of the developing paradigms in science, psychology, philosophy, spirituality, and art, has failed to point out one important fact: that the new consciousness will be the consciousness of a hearing people. We must therefore refine our hearing to the degree that it can effectively contribute to a breakthrough in consciousness. The purpose of the Yoga of Sound is to contribute to this evolution in consciousness by enhancing our cellular attunement to the rhythms of nature, aligning our own energy fields with those of the universe, and heightening our sensory faculties through intensified hearing abilities.

THE SPIRIT IS THE CONSCIOUS EAR

Dr. Alfred A. Tomatis, a revolutionary medical doctor and philosopher born in France, laid the groundwork for a new multidisciplinary science called Audio-Psycho-Phonology. His insights, which explain "the way we listen," have had a profound impact. In the early 1950s, Dr. Tomatis discovered that listening problems are the root cause of many learning problems.[2]

Tomatis began his work as an ear, nose, and throat specialist by trying to heal opera singers who had injured their hearing through the intensity of their own voice. His discovery that the voice can reflect the ear's ability to hear, a phenomenon known as the Tomatis Effect, is now applied in clinics worldwide to effectively treat a number of conditions, including autism and learning disabilities.[3] The Tomatis Effect complements the Sufi message of Hazrat Inayat Khan, which states that the human voice is a barometer of the human spirit, which in turn can be radically affected by working with the voice.

According to sound healer and educator Don Campbell, Tomatis's research defines the ear as a primary organ for multiple physical, emotional, and neurological development responses.[4] Tomatis discovered not only that the ear is to be credited for its complex ability to send information to the brain and the body (a task that is primary for hearing and sound perception), but also that our sense of hearing is crucial to our sense of balance and equilibrium.

The Tomatis method has proven that poor balance and difficulty in coordinating body movement can be rectified by correcting inconsistencies in the ear. The Tomatis method has also been successfully used to treat distractibility, restlessness, daydreaming, poor attention, and poor concentration in learning situations by rectifying inconsistencies in hearing. All these conditions can be considered symptomatic of listening problems, explains Campbell, because listening integrates sensations and perceptions.[5] In other words, hearing is crucial to the development and evolution of consciousness.

The ear training method of Tomatis is strikingly similar to the process of Hatha Yoga, which systematically works to increase physical balance and mental concentration through its postures. You may also want to recall the image of the ear proportioned by the golden mean discussed in chapter twelve as you read the following poem by Emily Dickinson:[6]

The Spirit is the Conscious Ear —
We actually Hear
When We inspect — that's audible —
That is admitted — Here —

For other Services — as Sound —
There hangs a smaller Ear
Outside the Castle — that Contain —
The other — only — Hear —

Interestingly, Tomatis titled his autobiography *The Conscious Ear: My Life of Transformation Through Listening.*[7]

WHAT IS CONSCIOUSNESS?

For thousands of years, the East has been preoccupied with consciousness. It is only now that Westerners are beginning to examine this fundamental quality in our own nature and in the universe. The West has always perceived God and Spirit as something separate from the world, separate from material existence. The East saw Spirit as consciousness, integral and intrinsic to all existence — material and nonmaterial — at every level of being. The deepest, or ultimate, plane is the realm of pure consciousness, pure spirit.

What happens when we start to take away our thoughts, our images, our concepts, our opinions, even our beliefs? What remains is consciousness. All our perceptions are just forms that our consciousness takes — appearances, so to speak. This has been the fundamental preoccupation of yoga: to eliminate the appearances, the illusion of maya, and discover the ultimate reality of Brahman, or pure consciousness.

Understanding Patanjali's statement that "yoga is the cessation of the modification and movements of the mind stuff" is the primary prerequisite to perceiving this pure consciousness. It clears the mirror. A parallel statement in Christianity is that of St. Paul: "Now we see clouded, as though in a mirror, but then [in the mystical state] we shall see face to face." This, too, is the perception of pure consciousness — except that consciousness is not a function of time. "Without moving," says the *Eesha Upanishad*, "the Spirit is everywhere." This means that wherever we go, wherever our body or mind travels, in waking or in dreaming, there our consciousness is. Even the biblical Psalmist prays:

Oh where can I hide from your spirit? From your presence, where can I flee?
If I ascend to the heavens, you are there; if I lie down in Sheol, you are there, too.
If I fly with the wings of dawn and alight beyond the sea,
Even there your hand will guide me, your right hand hold me fast.

Psalm 139

Our consciousness — from which we derive our identity, our sense of "I-ness" — is not dependent on space or time, explains Peter Russell, a physicist who has worked with Eastern philosophy and experimental psychology for several decades.[8] Consciousness begins with awareness: sensing our environment, sensing ourselves, sensing each other. Slowly we begin to sense the awareness of our being aware — not of something in particular, but the very awareness of awareness. This is the emergence of consciousness. This is when awareness is transformed into something deeper, fuller, and more independent.

Consciousness does not depend on an object. It simply is. The Hebrew name for God, "YHWH," means "I am that I am." This proclamation can be reflected infinitely as in facing mirrors: I am that I am that I am that I am... In other words, "I am consciousness." Consciousness has infinite depth, infinite height, infinite breadth, and infinite length. It proceeds infinitely inward and infinitely outward. The movements inherent within the vowels, as well as the streams of sacred sound that we have worked with, are essential to the expansion and development of our consciousness.

Consciousness is also timeless. "Before Abraham was, I am," said Jesus. Our normal experience of the passing of time is derived from change, explains Peter Russell.[9] The cycle of day and night, the beating of the heart, the passing of thoughts — all these reflect motions in time. Consciousness, on the other hand, is associated with our deepest sense of "I" and is eternal; it never changes. This deep identity of the true self, immersed in pure consciousness, is the objective of yoga practice.

The various forms of consciousness that we perceive as a result of our sensory experiences and our mental states — forms and patterns we identify with — are not our true, unchanging, eternal self. Each of these forms of consciousness has its own specific vibratory frequency. They are literally our personal "vibes," emanating from our core or simply orbiting our personal center. But pure consciousness transcends all attributes. It is that transpersonal presence of Nirguna Brahman — Spirit beyond all form or attribute. Eventually, when all form has been transformed, the pure form of consciousness remains. An ancient Zen koan asks the question: "If you blot out sense and sound, what do you hear?" The answer is samadhi, the vibration of pure consciousness.

SAMADHI: ESTABLISHING PURE CONSCIOUSNESS

THE WORD *sama* means "calm" or "tranquil." It is the state of mind personified by *dharma,* a harmony with all the laws of the universe. *Aadhi* means "primal." In other words, when action (karma) is in harmony with the laws of the universe, it becomes dharma, the universal code of truth. This is establishment in samadhi. Another interpretation of the word "samadhi" is that it is the primal, undisturbed state of the mind, free from all distractions and preoccupations. It is primordial union, perfect harmony with all that is, a goal to be realized by the yogi. The process of yoga is to still all the fluctuations of mind and body to reveal this primal state, which is always there, always present. Consciousness is often associated with light, just as sound is associated with matter. The Yoga of Sound, we can say, is the alchemical process of transforming matter into light, and incarnating light into matter.

Light, explains Peter Russell, is the sense of "I" that pervades our existence and that of every being on this planet; it is that common place from which we all derive our existence and identity, directly from the Divine, which is pure consciousness itself. This is why, at the deepest level of our existence, it is natural to feel so much in union (yoga) with pure consciousness, and why mystics around the world have proclaimed:

"I am God," "I am Brahman." This is not the individual human personality making the statement, but the knowledge of pure being that utters it. Samadhi is the state of being established in this deepest level of identity. There is no subject-object relationship here, as indicated by the following story. An amazing Jesuit priest by the name of Anthony De Mello once used it to explain the state of pure consciousness, or samadhi. I retell it with a Hindu flavor and in a way that applies directly to our Yoga of Sound process:

> *An old woman was seen going into a temple early each morning when the gates opened. Without budging even for a cup of water, she sat in front of the shrine all day, absorbed in deep meditation. Dutifully, she stood up at the last bell and walked out when the gates were about to be closed at night. The priest, somewhat curious, questioned her one day. "You seem to have a lot to talk to Shiva about," he prodded jokingly. The old woman looked deep and penetratingly into the* pujari's *eyes. "That's true," she replied. "But we're done talking in a couple of hours. At first I talk and Shiva listens. Later, Shiva speaks; I listen. As the day unfolds, neither of us speaks; we both listen. But as evening approaches, neither of us speaks, and neither of us listens."*

This is the process of sacred sound. It is a means of approaching the unknowable Brahman. Via sound, we progress through deeper levels of silence until we arrive at para, that level of sound where there is neither subject nor object. By persisting in our practice of the Yoga of Sound, we arrive at that place of pure consciousness. All obstructions have been burned up by the fire of our devotion and the power of our mantras. Consciousness alone remains.

BRAIN WAVES OF CONSCIOUSNESS

In 1908, an Austrian psychiatrist named Hans Berger discovered the existence of oscillating electrical waves in the brain. He named them "alpha" waves because they were the first electrical activity discovered in the brain. The publication of his findings in 1918 spurred an interest in these electrical waves. Early scientists mapped out different types of brain waves (alpha, beta, delta, and theta) and began to do psychophysical studies on the "natural reactivity" of these brain waves to sensory stimulation. None of these early investigators ever imagined that people could learn voluntary control of their own brain waves, which were thought to be an exclusively autonomic function. In 1962, with the emergence of biofeedback through a report of Dr. Joe Kamiya, the West discovered what yogis had known and practiced for thousands of years: that states of consciousness can be voluntarily induced.[10]

The four brain-wave states mapped out by scientists range from very rapid to very slow frequencies. In other words, the brain emits waves, and these frequencies are measured in hertz (Hz), or cycles per second. A normal person in the waking state generates beta waves of 13–30 Hz. This is our state of active awareness or active consciousness during our regular hours of work and play. When we are mentally awake and alert yet relaxed, we produce alpha waves in the range of 8–12 Hz. This is a coveted frequency range, as we are powerfully creative and productive in this state, drawing from a deep place of innate wisdom and limitless possibility.

When we sleep, we produce theta waves, from 3–7 Hz. An interesting meeting point is the alpha-theta range, a type of half-asleep, half-awake state — the type of consciousness that can also be induced by drugs such as LSD and MDMA (ecstasy). This amazing state of consciousness allows us to sense the energy of people and things fairly acutely.

The deepest level of consciousness mapped out by scientists is the delta state, an impressively slow frequency of 0.5–2 Hz. The brain goes into this wave pattern when a person is in a coma or suffering from a drug overdose. In other words, the delta state simulates a near-death experience. This state can also be temporarily produced by drugs such as sleeping pills and barbiturates.

These brain-wave states can be compared to the four states of consciousness symbolized by the mantra Om: waking, dreaming, deep sleep, and turiya. They can also be associated with the four stages of linguistic sound developed by the Vedic grammarians: vaikari, madhyama, pashyanti, and para. And we can seek to produce these states of consciousness through the four types of mantra utterances described by Tantric yogis: vacaka, upaamsu, maanasa, and tusnim. The deeper we get into the Yoga of Sound, the more realistic this possibility becomes — provided, of course, that we apply the methods properly.

Brain researchers also discovered that if the left ear is subjected to a specific frequency, say 400 Hz, and the right ear to a different one, say 410 Hz, the brain registers the difference between the two and emits a wave of the frequency that represents that difference (10 Hz, in this example). In other words, you can get your brain to emit specific waves and enter specific states of consciousness by pairing up sets of musical frequencies, a combination known as "binaural frequencies" or "binaural beats." This is what happens when we chant; the repetitive combinations of frequencies that make up the musical intervals of our chanting cause our brain to emit specific waves that deepen our states of consciousness.

The deeper we journey into ourselves using sound, the slower our brain waves become. The paradox is that instead of becoming dead to the world as our brain waves slow down, we awaken! We awaken to the true meaning and purpose of life, which is the experience of consciousness. Rather than fill ourselves with drugs that harm our body, mantras and musical tones can actually induce states of consciousness that propagate self-realization and samadhi. It's a cheaper, safer, decidedly organic way to alter consciousness. This is the ultimate benefit of Yoga of Sound practice: it is an alchemy of the soul.

SPIRITUAL PROGRESS: THE EVOLUTION OF CONSCIOUSNESS

Progress along the spiritual path is best measured in terms of consciousness, which becomes more refined, heightened, spacious, deep, full, and rich as we journey inward. An evolved consciousness also contains all the spiritual qualities we admire: peace, love, joy, freedom, confidence, connectedness, integrity, wholeness, and abundance. Although the word "consciousness" is often used interchangeably with "awareness," I would like to contrast these two terms to help define this fifth element of Sound Yoga.

Spiritual practice *begins* with awareness, but it should lead to consciousness. Awareness is the individual self sensing an objective reality. Consciousness, on the other hand, is the very substratum of all existence; it is intrinsically self-aware. Awareness is dualistic: "I am aware of something." Consciousness simply is; it is nondualistic and all-pervasive, as in "I am." Awareness is partial; when we are aware of something, our perception singles out that object from other things. Consciousness is complete and inclusive; it is a sense of the whole, all parts included.

You can be "aware" without fully developing your consciousness; you can sense something without realizing its complete significance. Consciousness, on the other hand, includes awareness, intelligence, perception, and the ability to respond creatively on behalf of a larger body. In consciousness, awareness becomes cosmic; all its components function on behalf of a collective whole.

Spiritual practice should always be undertaken on behalf of the whole. That is why the systematic development of consciousness is essential to spirituality.

YOGA NIDRA: REFINING YOUR CONSCIOUSNESS

FOR THOUSANDS of years, yogis have practiced *yoga nidra,* a healing and spiritually nourishing exercise that can significantly alter our brainwave patterns and take us to the realm of pure consciousness. In this state, the body is able to renew itself spiritually and energetically, and you can see your way through complex problems — be they spiritual, personal, or work-related — and then return to your life with renewed spirit and confidence.

Although yoga nidra may be practiced at any time of day or night, it is best to perform it when you are relaxed and alert. We often forget the value of proper relaxation, which actually increases our productivity and helps us achieve more by allowing us to expend less energy. In the following exercise, we will use the word "awareness" to help us progress toward a heightened consciousness. Eventually, both words will point to the same experience.

Acute listening, feeling, and receptivity are the objective of yoga nidra. Through this exercise, we learn to hear and feel the vibrations of our body and our mind, not just with our physical ears but also with our spiritual ears, our intuition, and the deepest sensitivities of our soul.

To perform yoga nidra, make sure that you are wearing loose-fitting clothing, preferably without underwear. The ideal is to wear no clothing — just being clothed with the sky.

Going Downstream

1. Lie down in the corpse position, savasana, and allow a deep letting-go to take place. This means that we don't push anything out of our awareness, nor do we encourage anything to remain in our field of sensing. Allow your awareness to pass into the region of your head and sense your eyes, nose, mouth, ears, and cheeks, and the sides, top, and back of your head. Stay aware of all sensations, whether pleasant or unpleasant. This is a bit like taking stock of your inventory without making plans about what you are going to do with it.

   As you take stock, allow your thinking mind and your imagination to rest without judgment or commentary; observe any visual manifestations of energy in each region you explore. Generally, your sensations may appear as images, colors, shapes, or patterns in your mind's eye. Also stay attuned to sonic manifestations of energy, which may take the form of words, sounds, rhythms, or vibratory textures.

2. Shift your awareness smoothly from your head to your throat, and practice the same totality of awareness. Feel the texture of energy caused by the passage of air in your throat, and deliberately regulate its flow by performing the audible breath. Make sure your face stays relaxed as you perform this subtly controlled breathing, allowing a steady stream of energy to flow in and out of your body.

3. Let go of the controlled, audible breathing and move your awareness into your chest and solar plexus. Isolate your breathing to your upper chest by keeping your stomach relaxed. Gradually settle down in your heart-space and stay visually present to all manifestations of energy in your chest region. Keep your mind free of all deliberate activity as you listen intently to all the sounds that register, such as your pulse and heartbeat.

4. Isolate your breathing to your lower lungs, around your abdomen; your mid-chest and upper chest should stay

relaxed. Observe the inflation and deflation of your abdomen as you continue to breathe this way for a short while. Inhale deeply into your lower lungs and hold the breath inside for a moment; release the breath slowly, relaxing your body and allowing your awareness to descend into your pelvis and genital region. Relax your upper, middle, and lower lungs and try to isolate your breathing to the region just above your pelvic area. Observe the effects of this type of breathing around your genitals, and stay aware of the sensations that register there. Be present to any pulsations, images, or sounds as they manifest in and around your sex organs.

5. Move your awareness down farther, into the base of your spinal column, and become aware of your anal opening. Gently contract and relax the anal sphincter muscles (performing the *ashwini mudra;* see appendix two), which you can work in rhythm with your breath or at whatever pace is comfortable for you. After a while, let go of these contractions and move your awareness into your thighs; stay present to all the sensations in your upper legs. Slowly move into your calves, then your ankles, and eventually rest your awareness in your feet; stay present to the sensations in your toes and the soles of your feet. Allow your entire body to sink into the floor and merge with the energy of the earth (or whatever material you are lying on).

Upstream and Downstream, in Your Nightgown

In the reverse process, you will keep your entire body relaxed; there will be no controlled activity of breath or muscle. We will use the word "consciousness" instead of "awareness" from this moment onward. While earlier you might have felt somewhat removed from your sensations, everything you will now experience will feel grounded and much more immediate to your sensing.

1. FEET TO HEAD: Starting with the feet, slowly allow your consciousness to creep up your legs, feeling the heaviness of your muscles as though something is gently pushing through

you, like a serpent entering your body. This experience may take a visual form, such as smoke or a golden glow that makes its way up your body. Direct your consciousness slowly and deliberately up your body until it reaches the top of your head, allowing it to penetrate every cell and tissue in its path. The movement of your consciousness is accentuated by the stillness of your body. When you arrive at your head, stay there and take in all the sensations manifesting in your head, as you did when you started this practice.

2. HEAD TO FEET: Journey downward into your throat and toward your feet without controlling your breathing in any way. Keep still and relaxed; allow your body to breathe naturally while your consciousness explores each region. Don't spend too much time in one place, but don't spend too little time, either. Above all, don't skip over a region.

3. UP AND DOWN: Journey consciously from your feet to your head, but do it a little faster, making sure you aren't going faster than will allow you to take in all the energy and sensations you are encountering on your path. Travel up and down your body a few times as fast as is comfortable for you. Your speed should match your consciousness in one smooth process.

4. REST: Eventually, come to rest. Choose a point of reference in your body, such as the movement of your abdomen, your heartbeat, or the delicate sensation of your breath in your nostrils. Keep your mind free from deliberate thoughts or images, but don't suppress what naturally arises. Refrain from following ideas or feeding images that pop up; stay attuned to all that is going on in the entire field of energy that is your body.

5. BRINGING CLOSURE: When you are ready to emerge from this experience, initiate movement in your body. Start by flexing your toes. Then move your feet and shake your legs gently without disturbing the upper part of your body. Next, flex your fingers and hands; shake your arms and

forearms lightly. Finally, move your head slowly from side to side, then stretch your whole body any way you feel inclined to. Roll over onto your left side, and use your right hand to raise yourself up in a way that minimizes pressure on your spine. (You can reverse this process if you are left-handed.)

6. Sit quietly for a few minutes before you resume normal activities.

THE REALIZATION OF CONSCIOUSNESS

SELF-REALIZATION and consciousness are to the East what love and justice are to the West. The realization of consciousness is the realization of our immortality; it is what remains after death. The Indian mystic Kabir urges us: "Oh Friend! Hope for the Divine whilst you live, know whilst you live, understand whilst you live; for in life deliverance abides."[11] Matter, life, energy, and intelligence are ultimately consciousness; the whole purpose of the Yoga of Sound is to realize the fullness of this consciousness. This depth of consciousness is available to us, right here and right now, in this body, in this life, in this world.

This is full, that is full
From fullness, fullness proceeds
Taking fullness away from fullness
Fullness alone remains.

Poor-na-ma-da-ha, Poor-nam-idam
Poor-naat, Poor-nam Udach-ya-te
Poor-nas-ya, Poor-na-maa-daa-ya
Poor-nam-eva, Ava-shish-ya-te

From the *Vedas*

PART 5

INTEGRATION

LIVING THE LIFE OF A SOUND YOGI

The little space within the heart is as great as a vast universe.
The heavens and the earth are there, and the sun,
and the moon, and the stars; fire and lightning and winds
are there; and all that now is and all that is not: for the whole
universe is Him and He dwells within our heart.

The Chandogya Upanishad[1]

CHAPTER 17

LIVING THE YOGA OF SOUND

Combining all the elements of the Yoga of Sound into a regular practice requires treating the process like a garden. Prepare the soil with the elements of Sound Yoga, then plant your mantras. In this chapter, I will outline suggestions for creating a living, breathing practice of Sound Yoga.

When you first start out, a spiritual practice is fragile. You must tend to your fledgling practices regularly and ensure that they are given sufficient sunlight, water, and nourishment. The spotlight of your consciousness, the water of your breath, and the nourishment of devotion will care for this garden of your soul. Some saplings may need protection from overexposure, so practice moderation; that is the true spirit of yoga.

Becoming excessively preoccupied with the world and losing perspective in relation to our spiritual goals is normal. It's a sort of temporary spiritual amnesia. During such periods, we may neglect our garden, allowing weeds to grow in our absence. Meister Eckhart once said: "It is not so much that God does not dwell within us; it is we who have gone out for a walk." When you return home, tend to your garden again; through your loving attentiveness, revive the beauty and harmony you enjoyed before.

Attending workshops and retreats, reading new books, and listening to new music are all ways of visiting other gardens; we learn from these experiences and bring back new flowers to plant in our own garden. It is also helpful to study privately with experts. They show us how to landscape our garden, and they help us discover new vistas and paths, sometimes pointing out rare and exotic flowers we didn't know existed in our own backyard.

THE VALUE OF AN INTEGRATED SOUND YOGA

Our choices of specific mantras and exercises from among the various sound streams may vary according to our moods, character, and circumstances. Each stream can perform particular functions in our lives, responding to specific problems and challenges we face. An integrated practice that maintains all four streams is ideal. When I first came to the United States, I found life here to be full of stress, with financial burdens, legal responsibilities, and work competition. I found that Vedic mantras and the practice of Shabda Yoga offered me strength and protection through their articulate sounds, often preventing me from feeling vulnerable when preparing for my day's tasks or when going through difficult negotiations in my life. These practices were particularly powerful during legal battles, dealing with insurance companies, and other similar situations. The Vedic mantras further enabled me to develop effective communication skills, building confidence and maturity into my speaking voice. As a bonus, they added great texture to my singing voice!

I was also deeply troubled, when I moved to the West, by our lack of connection with nature here. We wear mostly synthetic clothes, eat unwholesome foods, move about with extremely rapid methods of transportation, and rely too much on technology to artificially control our environments. All of this severs our connection with nature, often leading to poor health and even disease. In response, I have found that the use of Tantric mantras and the practices of Shakti Yoga help me maintain an intimate relationship with my physical body and my sensuality, removing blocks and constrictions that obstruct the optimal flow of energy in my nervous system. This ancient knowledge has been utilized for many thousands of years, and it costs us nothing. Why not put it to the test and give it a chance?

Even though the West is a culture that loves community effort and teamwork, it often lacks true and consistent emotional fulfillment. A pervasive loneliness and isolation invariably seeks to fulfill itself in superficial relationships or unhealthy sexual obsessions. In my daily practice, Bhava Yoga mantras help release love and devotion in my heart, providing me with a deep, expansive emotional fulfillment. Bhava Yoga also helps regulate my emotions, staving off manic highs and crushing lows. I am grateful to have an extraordinary companion in my wife Asha, but without the devotional mantras we both employ in our spiritual practice, our relationship would be very different; it would lack the luster and vibrancy we've become accustomed to.

Through Nada Yoga, we can fine-tune our bodies and our minds to resonate with the harmony in all of creation, from atoms and cells to flowers and planets. We are surrounded by music in our culture, but most of it does little to help us on the soul level of our being. Through Nada Yoga meditations, we develop insight into the true nature of music, effortlessly tapping the healing power of sound and becoming better equipped to attune ourselves to the varying circumstances in our lives. Listening keenly to others and to ourselves enables us to choose what is good and stay away from that which is harmful. As a result, we enjoy greater empathy in our relationships and enhanced satisfaction in our work, and we contribute a more pleasing vibration to the energy of our societies. This is the fruit of the Yoga of Sound.

THE YOGA OF SOUND FOR BUSY PEOPLE

THE WONDERFUL THING about the Yoga of Sound is that you can start anywhere, then keep adding layers of depth and skill to even the simplest exercises. You can also practice Sound Yoga for relatively short periods, depending on what your schedule allows, and still enjoy many of its benefits. The charm of this tradition is that we are inspired to use sound to affect our consciousness and that of others almost all the time.

If you are busy — as most of us are — I recommend that you distribute your practice among four segments of the day: morning, noon, evening, and night. Choose one of the following options:

MINIMUM: 5 minutes per segment = 20 minutes per day

MODERATE: 15 minutes per segment = 1 hour per day

IDEAL: 21 minutes per segment = 1 hour and 24 minutes per day

We can also combine the various Yoga of Sound streams into a daily practice. I recommend Shabda Yoga in the morning, shortly after you wake up; Shakti Yoga around noon, just before lunch; Bhava Yoga in the evening, after you return from work; and Nada Yoga at night, preferably just before you go to sleep. This strategy allows the key principles of each of these streams of sacred sound to work when people most need them during the day. You may also use any of the practices from any of the streams, combining them during any time of the day or night, depending on what you need and how you need it.

Daily Practice

Morning: Shabda Yoga

I SUGGEST Shabda Yoga in the morning because it helps prepare you for the day ahead; it fortifies your soul against the challenges you have to face. This stream of Sound Yoga is best practiced twenty minutes after you wake up, allowing enough time for you to be fully alert during your practice. Regular spiritual practice and an enhanced vocabulary of mantras can help you deal effectively with issues so that they don't become problems. I recommend, therefore, that you use a combination of Vedic mantras (appendix one) and positive affirmations at the start of your day. The great yogic breath, along with sectional breathing (see chapter thirteen for both techniques), is also helpful in the morning.

Noon: Shakti Yoga

SHAKTI YOGA practices are fantastic for dealing with energy bleeds that can take place at work. Around noon, or just before you eat your lunch, take stock of the most powerful experiences you've had that morning. Pay close attention to the effect those situations have had on your energy centers. Notice whether any of your chakras are blocked. Use shakti mantras and the alternate-nostril breathing *nadi sodhana* (appendix four) to clear these blockages. As you build up your vocabulary in this stream of Sound Yoga, you may introduce other practices as well.

Evening: Bhava Yoga

Bhava Yoga is best saved for evening. After we finish our day's work, we can look forward to a wonderful experience of union when we return home. For those who work at home, this is the ideal resolution at the end of the day. Light a lamp, burn a stick of incense, and chant devotionally for five to seven minutes; often, that's all it takes to bring a sense of completion to your day. Chant to Jesus, to Ram, to Krishna, or to the Buddha. Pour out your heart to the Divine, and offer everything — the positive and the not-so-positive. Trust that it will all be better tomorrow. After this, you can give yourself fully to your lover, yourself, your friends, or your community, depending on what you have planned for that evening.

Night: Nada Yoga

At night, before you go to bed, sit quietly and attune yourself to everything that has transpired during the day. Let it all pass through you and out of you. Practice yoga nidra (see chapter sixteen) and attune your body to the Divine presence so that you can sleep peacefully in the Divine embrace. Pay attention to your breathing, and try to remain conscious as you enter into sleep. You will find yourself well-rested in the morning.

FORTIFYING YOUR PRACTICE YEAR-ROUND

DAILY: Keep a Yoga of Sound journal to make brief notes on the insights or challenges that present themselves to you on your journey. Value the process; it is your best teacher.

WEEKLY: Once a week, spend an hour learning new mantras and musical intervals. Introduce them in your practice during the rest of the week. Use about fifteen minutes of this hour to prolong your meditative awareness and center deeply in the experience. Review your journal notes and mark important entries.

MONTHLY: Once a month, take a two- or three-hour mini-workshop, or schedule a private session with an expert to improve your skills in Sound Yoga. Otherwise, design your own private mini-retreat by concentrating on a specific breathing practice, mantra, or movement; seek to enter more fully into the tradition. Review the marked entries in your journal and summarize your progress in a brief comment.

QUARTERLY: Once every quarter, take a one-day (five-to-eight-hour) retreat. You can do this in your own home, at a retreat center, or in an isolated cabin by the sea. Ensure that you will not be disturbed, and that it is okay for you to use vocal sound in the place where you are on retreat. Immerse yourself in the experience; review all the practices you know and evaluate them. Reflect on key journal entries you've made related to this discipline. Review your monthly comments and write a brief, single-paragraph description of your progress.

ANNUALLY: If you have the time and resources, take a weeklong workshop or retreat on the Yoga of Sound once every year. This will give you new insights into the tradition. Review your quarterly descriptions and write a half-page summary of what you have assimilated during the past year. Title your summary, including the year it refers to. Use the second half of the page to project what you would like to assimilate during the coming year. Title and date this section, too.

EVERY THREE TO SEVEN YEARS: Go on a pilgrimage. This could be to a sacred spot within your own country or overseas. Pilgrimage is a form of deep soul cleansing, enabling us to start anew with a fresh perspective. My wife and I go on a group pilgrimage every year to holy temples in South India. This is the Hindu way, which sees life itself as a pilgrimage, a passage through this plane toward ultimate fulfillment. You are always welcome to join us, or you may plan your own experience.

SIMPLE WAYS TO KEEP THE EXPERIENCE ALIVE

THE SHOWER: When you start your day, devote at least a few minutes to chanting reverently in the shower. Place your palms together and chant some mantras as you attune yourself to the sound of the flowing water. This will help cleanse your mind while your body is being cleansed.

WALKING: When you walk down the street, chant rhythmically to the sound of your breathing. Find a mantra that complements your pace and energy at that time. This will put joy into your step and generate beneficial chemicals in your brain.

EXERCISE WORKOUT: Chant before and after your exercise or yoga workout. You can do this internally if you're in a public place. It will connect you more intimately with your body and help you stay more present to the physiological changes that are occurring.

THE COMPUTER: At work, sit quietly in front of your computer before you start the workday. Mentally recite a mantra or a series of mantras for one minute; this will clear your mind and help you function more efficiently. Do the same thing before you leave your workstation. Even half a minute will help configure your computer with positive energy and encourage you to enjoy returning to it.

BATHROOM BREAK: When you take a bathroom break, use mantras to occupy your mind for a full minute before, after, or even during your time on the toilet. If you have the whole bathroom to yourself, lock the door, stand with your feet and palms together (with clean hands), face the door, and chant for a full minute. Harmonize the flow of your breathing, then step out peacefully and confidently.

TRAFFIC SIGNALS: At a traffic signal, chant quietly and breathe evenly; visualize the road to your destination as a smooth flow of energy toward its source. Fill the interior of your vehicle with positive sound vibrations. If you are in gridlock, chant aloud and listen to the sound of your mantras filling your car; you might want to close the windows to keep the energy contained.

BUSINESS MEETINGS: Chant internally as you enter the room. Make eye contact and smile while continuing to chant mentally; this will help you awaken the best in people and in yourself. If you find knots developing against your spine during the discussions, regulate your breathing with the sectional breathing or the complete breath (see chapter thirteen). This will enable you to listen more attentively and communicate more effectively.

LOVEMAKING: Chant internally or, even better, chant with your lover for a full minute. You will engage each other in an authentic way afterward, as the chanting will disperse any negative energy or expectations. Regulate your breathing while engaged in the act; it will smoothen and enhance the process. Play a CD of chanting in the background to channel your energy differently. I've gotten very affirming reports about my own recordings, by the way — particularly *P.M. Yoga Chants.*

OPENING YOUR MAIL: Place your palms on your mail bundle and chant a mantra three times before you start opening your mail. This will help you stay detached from outcomes and embrace whatever is being placed before you in life.

TRANSIT AND TRAVEL: Lounges, trains, airports, airplanes, and even sitting rooms are great places to attune your energy to the Divine presence. Chant your mantra internally; even half a minute will help you center deeply and cause your energy to flow optimally through your nervous system.

COMBINATIONS AND SEQUENCES

Treat the Yoga of Sound as an organic process that will keep unfolding as you get into it more deeply. The secret is to learn each principle, mantra, and technique so well that you can combine them in energetic sequences that are just right for you in a given moment, or for a particular phase in your life. Such combinations must be seamless. As a reference, I've provided you with some simple examples. You can substitute your own choice of mantra if you don't feel inspired by the one recommended. I know this sounds a bit like a menu, but a menu is a good analogy, since mantras are food for the soul.

Morning Combinations

1. Stand in the posture of prayer, prathanaasana (see chapter twelve), and loudly recite the mantra *Asa-ṯo Ma Saḏ-ga-ma-ya; Ṯa-ma-so Ma Jyo-ṯir-ga-ma-ya; Mriṯ-yor Ma A-mri-ṯam-ga-ma-ya.* Draw from the articulate power of shabda to manifest the best outcomes in your life. You may then perform Zikr (body turning; see chapter fifteen) in silence, and later lie

down in the corpse pose (see chapter twelve) to use the mantra *So-Ham*.

2. Sit in vajrasana (between your heels). If you notice blockage in your system, perform the sectional breathing practices, then conclude by chanting the mantra *Om* while doing the great yogic breath (chapter thirteen).

3. Sit in your meditation position and chant the mantra *Kra-to Sma-ra Kru-tam Sma-ra*. Follow this with the alternate nostril breathing (nadi sodhana; see appendix four), and end with cranial buzzing (brahmari mudra; see appendix four), performed with the six-way seal (see appendix four).

Midday Combinations

1. Sit in your meditation position and go through all the chakra bijas (see appendix two). Perform each bija three times and visualize energy opening each chakra as you chant the appropriate mantra. After the chanting, stay attuned to the physical experience of each chakra region in your body.

2. Go through all the vowels and their movements, as described in "Dancing the Vowels" (chapter fifteen). Repeat the exercise by riding the sounds on your breath. Conclude with sounding them internally.

3. Find a quiet, isolated spot, preferably outdoors. Chant one of the deity bijas (appendix two) for one full minute. Sit quietly and pay attention to your breathing, then perform nadi sodhana, the alternate nostril breathing (see appendix four).

Evening Combinations

1. Perform the bhava yoga ritual (see chapter nine), then sit quietly in meditation for a minute. You may put together the ingredients for the ritual by buying flowers on the way home from work, or you may perform the ritual mentally, as described in manasika puja (see chapter nine).

2. Stand in the prayer posture (see chapter twelve) for a minute, then launch into the Zikr (see chapter nine), using the mantra

Om–Eeshaa–Vaasyam–Idham. Sink into savasana, the corpse pose (see chapter twelve), and place your attention on the delicate sensation of breath passing through your nostrils.

3. Do a meditation walk (see chapter fifteen) while mindfully, rhythmically chanting the mantra *Hare Raama, Hare Raama – Raama Raama, Hare Hare – Hare Krishna, Hare Krishna – Krishna Krishna, Hare Hare*. Then find a quiet spot under a tree and perform the great yogic breath (chapter thirteen).

Night Combinations

1. Lie in the corpse position (see chapter twelve) and chant the mantra *Shree Ram – Jai Ram – Jai Jai Ram* for a few minutes. Touch parts of your body, reciting mantras to consecrate your body before going to bed.
2. Perform the yoga nidra exercise (chapter sixteen), but don't run your awareness up and down your body rapidly, as it would keep you awake. Mentally chant long *Om* mantras that continue internally over many breaths. Your consciousness will expand dramatically while you sleep.
3. Sit in vajrasana, between your heels. Perform the six-way seal (*shanmukhi mudra,* or *yoni mudra;* see appendix four), but without the buzzing. Then rest your awareness on the motion of your abdomen. Later, lie facing the ground turning your head to the right, pressing your left ear against your left arm using your arm as a headrest. Keep your right ear wide open and listen intently to the sounds of the night.

Create your own sequences, and don't judge them harshly. No one else can ever come close to the music that you yourself are hearing and creating. You must put the notes together, hold the baton in your hand, and conduct the orchestra of your own personality.

There is no guarantee that a fixed sequence will always bring you the same result because everything about you is constantly changing: the food you ate, an argument, a problem at work, and the position of your body as you slept — all affect you in this moment. You will change after your next meal, or as soon as you and your lover kiss and make up. As you continue to expand your mantra vocabulary, enter deeply into the elements of SoundYoga and develop an integrated practice using the various streams of sacred sound. Over time, your sequences will become more and more like a well-made film, with superb cinematography, seamless segues, and an excellent sound track. Good luck, and have fun along the way.

EPILOGUE

The benefits of science and technology — high-fidelity sound systems, advanced audio recording processes, and the convenience of car stereos, boom boxes, and portable music systems — can all be used to enhance our spiritual practice, enabling us to channel consciousness in ways never before experienced. The Yoga of Sound can play an important role in this era, bridging the gap between the human and technological realms by employing the living power of the human voice and the resonant temple of the human body.

I like to picture Shabda Yoga harnessing huge swirling vortexes of cosmic energy as it expands infinitely; Shakti Yoga stepping this energy down to function in our body through the chakras; Bhava Yoga receiving the finest and purest form of energy as it spirals directly into the core of our being; and Nada Yoga sustaining the entire experience in one harmonious balance.

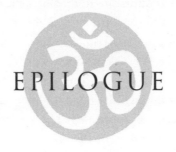

The Yoga of Sound is, I believe, the next step in spirituality. I'm not just referring to the Hindu traditions that form the foundation of what we've explored in this book. I am excited about all the global explorations of sonic spirituality and consciousness. I believe that musicians and music producers are our new priests and shamans; performances are our greatest rituals; and lyrical expressions are our most popular mantras, as they echo through the minds of listeners around the world.

Something powerful is happening. The evolutionary process has been stepped up to new and dramatic levels; with this, of course, comes the danger of self-annihilation, since only a portion of the human population has found its way to the mouth of the spiritual birth canal. Others feel the passage but are unable to see how things can change, while mother Gaia groans in travail. She is not as healthy as she used to be, and as we struggle to be born into a new consciousness, we may hurt both ourselves and the mother who is giving birth to us.

AMERICA: BIRTHING GROUND FOR A NEW CIVILIZATION

During the Vedic period in India, the Aryan integration into Harrappan culture was violent and oppressive. It developed the skin-color caste system that has been the bane of Hindu society for thousands of years. The dark-skinned Dravidians, the original inhabitants of the land, were subjugated even as their mathematics and other advanced knowledge were being harnessed by the established Aryan state. Despite these conditions, the Vedic culture and religion that emerged in India between 1500 B.C. and 500 B.C. developed into one of the most powerful spiritual traditions on the planet.

I believe that we can draw an analogy between that tumultuous period of racial convergence in ancient India and the current convergence of diverse cultural and religious streams here in America. Indeed, this second convergence may turn out to be far more pronounced than what took place on the Indian subcontinent 3,500 years ago. It may even officially usher in the second Axial period, when the many and the One come together in the All. The present conditions are more democratic, with healthier checks and balances, a more developed human species, and an extraordinary amount of information available to anyone seeking it. The signs point to a new civilization being born here in America; in the words of Wayne Teasdale, we hope that it will be "a civilization with a heart."[1]

America is obviously a fledgling culture — just a few hundred years old, in comparison to the thousand-year histories of other cultures — and it frightens the rest of the world that this culture has the technological power to destroy life on earth. But the opposite is equally true: America has the potential to turn inward and discover its spiritual power to become the protector and nurturer of the world. There is no doubt that Americans are a deeply spiritual people. Despite a cultural tendency toward superficiality, Americans are eager to learn new things and willing to give untried ideas a chance. This refreshing eagerness has drawn, and continues to draw, many spiritual teachers from around the world, contributing to a unique perspective enriched by diverse and profound worldviews.

But there is also a shadow here in America: a history of racial prejudice that continues to assert itself along with the development of corporate greed that cares nothing for the global human family. To our credit, this shadow is dying. In the midst of the mass mentality of obsessive consumerism, a spiritual force is gathering momentum in America. Many spiritual teachers have pointed to the attacks of September 11 as precipitating a spiritual awakening of immense magnitude. This evolutionary process is now pushing global consciousness through the spiritual birth canal, and each of us must play our part in ushering in our own new life.

TIME TO TAKE FLIGHT

My hope is that yogis and spiritual seekers in America will earnestly take up the study and practice of the Yoga of Sound; I truly believe that it can contribute an essential element to the spiritual depth that people are seeking. Americans have a natural openness to absorbing information and are good at developing teaching systems once they have learned a practice; they also know how to propagate their knowledge effectively to the rest of the world.

As I said earlier, although there is already a wonderful flowering of interest in Sound Yoga, this interest has placed too much emphasis on Bhakti Yoga mantras, and not enough on Tantric and Vedic mantras. These two latter streams are generally not being practiced or taught skillfully enough to communicate the true power and potency of mantras. By incorporating Vedic and Tantric mantras into your yoga practice and your daily prayers and rituals, you will discover for yourself the vision of India's Rishis, those enlightened individuals who authored the *Vedas,* the *Upanishads,* and the *Bhagavad Gita*. Once discovered, this vision will find a new and exciting articulation in our mix of cultures and perspectives.

For the past few decades, yoga has been presented to Americans free of its mystical and cultural traditions in order to make it appear safe and acceptable. This has eased its entry into the mainstream of American culture, precluding opposition from religious groups and establishing credibility with the medical profession. However, now that both Western medicine and Western religion are gravitating toward yoga, I feel that it is time for American yogis and spiritual practitioners to reintroduce the yoga of sacred sound. Such a study will empower the American soul, infusing the growing practice of yoga in this country with a mystical system for reaching the highest goal of samadhi. This will allow American yoga practice — both on and off the mat — to reach new levels of spiritual achievement. Perhaps it was part of the Divine plan that the physical emphasis on Hatha Yoga in the West has tempered our spiritual and nervous systems, preparing people to efficiently handle the energy that mantras are capable of releasing. The chariot is ready; it is now time for the soul to take flight.

> *Know the Atman [the Spirit] as the Lord of the chariot, and the body as the chariot itself.*
> *Know that reason is the charioteer, and the mind indeed is the reins.*
> *The horses, they say, are the senses, and their paths are the objects of sense.*
> *The [person] whose chariot is driven by reason, who watches and holds the reins of the mind, reaches the end of the journey, the supreme everlasting Spirit.*
>
> **Katha Upanishad**[2]

*OM TAT SAT**

* This pithy statement, often used to conclude spiritual discourses and mantra chanting, translates as: "Om. That's the truth." On a humorous note, it actually sounds like, "Om, that's it!"

APPENDIX 1

SHABDA YOGA: VEDIC MANTRAS

PRONUNCIATION

Applying some simple pronunciation techniques will bring the practice of mantra closer to your body and help activate the intended experience of the mantra. I have avoided using standard diacritical marks; many people don't use them properly, and others find them complicated.

I have also introduced pronunciation gradually, instead of all at once, so that you can progress one mantra at a time, employing the rules you know and learning new ones as you go along. The accompanying audio tracks will further assist you with the pronunciation of several mantras.

The chanting of Shabda mantras should be commanding, precise, and articulate. Adding a devotional quality and intention to these mantras is recommended, but this should always be done without sacrificing their articulate power.

A VEDIC MANTRA TO GUIDE US ON THE PATH TO ENLIGHTENMENT

The following mantra is to be used before meditation, yoga practice, or any spiritual undertaking. It is best used in the morning, shortly after awakening:

Asa-to Ma Sad-ga-ma-ya.
Ta-ma-so Ma Jyo-tir-ga-ma-ya.
Mrit-yor Ma A-mri-tam-ga-ma-ya.

Translation: Lead me from the unreal to the real, from darkness to light, from death to immortality.

Notes on pronunciation: Underlined letters indicate placing the tip of the tongue gently against a slightly open set of teeth: *t* sounds like the "th" in *thick; d* sounds like "th" in *there.*

The *r* is rolled on the roof of the palate — toward the front — like the Spanish "r." Try placing the tip of your tongue on the roof of your mouth behind your upper teeth and vibrating it on your upper palate. Note: By contrast, the American "r" is more in the center of the mouth's roof and pronounced without using the tip of the tongue.

Prolonged vowels are written twice: "aa" is a long-sounding "aah," double the sounding of a regular "a." Avoid excessive extension of double vowels.

- *a* is pronounced "ah," as in "father"
- *o* is pronounced as in "omen"
- *u* is pronounced as in "who" but without aspiration.

There are two vowels to watch out for:

- *e* is pronounced like the "a" in "acorn"
- *i* is pronounced like "ee," as in "feet"

Example: *Om Ma-ni Pad-me Hoom* would be pronounced "Om Mah-knee Padh-may Whom." Capital letters will help you identify individual words within the mantric sequence, and hyphens separate the syllables to assist in pronunciation.

Tones for the Mantra

ANY COMFORTABLE TONE can serve as your base pitch, or fundamental. The high tone above it should be just slightly higher, the low tone moderately lower. In the morning, a half tone above and a whole tone below are recommended (example: C, C sharp, B-flat). For the evening, a whole tone above and a whole tone below the fundamental are suggested (example: C, D, B-flat). Read them from left to right, like a line of music.

HIGH			*Ma*			*ma*	
BASE		*to*			*ga*		*ya*
LOW	*Asa*			*Sad*			

HIGH			*Ma*			*ga ma*	
BASE		*so*			*tir*		*ya*
LOW	*Ta ma*			*Jyo*			

HIGH			*Ma*			*ga ma*	
BASE		*yor*			*tam*		*ya*
LOW	*Mrit*			*A mri*			

THE SACRED GAYATRI TO ILLUMINATE OUR MEDITATIONS

This mantra is known as the mother of the Vedas. It is whispered into the ears of every orthodox Hindu boy who comes of age and is to be instructed in the spiritual life. The Gayatri is to be used at least three times in succession; 108 times each day is traditional. It is most effective at dawn and at dusk. Use this mantra to celebrate the power of the Divine in sound and in light, drawing into your soul the illuminatory power of spiritual awakening.

Om Bhur Bhu-vas Su-va-ha
Tat Sa-vi-tur Va-re ń-yam
Bhar-go De-vas-ya Dhi-ma-hi
Dhi-yo-yo-nah Pra-cho-da-yaat

Translation: Salutations to that sacred sound present in the earth, the heavens, and that which is beyond. May the glorious splendor of that Divine life illuminate our meditation.

Notes on pronunciation: In this mantra, you will encounter hard consonants. Any consonant with an "h" beside it indicates that it is aspirated (pronounced while breathing out).

The *bhu* is pronounced like slurring "boohoo" into a single-syllable "bhoo." Say it like you want to playfully scare someone!

I have changed the traditional spelling of *Sva-ha* to *Su-va-ha* to reflect the proper pronunciation of this word when chanted.

Remember the underlined *t* and *d* as in the previous mantra.

n (in *Varenyam)* is pronounced by curling the tongue upward, into the middle of the upper palate, like "n" in the word "earn."

The underlined *dh* has the tip of the tongue between the teeth but pronounced with a lot of emphasis.

The underlined *n* places the tip of your tongue very lightly against the teeth. That's how *namaste* should be pronounced. Notice how your tongue is positioned at the end of the word "teeth;" say the letter *n* in that position, and you will understand how to pronounce this particular *n*.

The *ch* is like the "ch" in "cheap." *(Pra-cho-da-yaat)*

Tones for the Mantra

HIGH				*va*	
BASE	*Om Bhur Bhu*		*Su*		*ha*
LOW		*vas*			

HIGH		*Sa*				*re n*	
BASE	*Tat*			*tur*	*Va*		*yam*
LOW			*vi*				

HIGH		*go*			*ya*			
BASE	*Bhar*			*vas*		*Dhi*	*ma*	*hi*
LOW			*De*					

HIGH				*nah*				*a*	
BASE	*Dhi*		*yo*		*Pra*		*da ya*		*t*
LOW		*yo*				*cho*			

A VEDIC MANTRA TO HEAL OUR PLANET

THIS MANTRA is an eloquent yogic prayer that treats the whole world as our own body. At this time in history, when our planet is being ravaged by industrial exploitation and sickened by voluminous quantities of toxic waste, this prayer is especially appropriate. Chant it at least once a day; thrice in succession is preferable. Whenever possible, chant it with a group.

Lo-kah Sa-mas-ta Sukhi-no Bha-van-tu

Translation: May our world be established with well-being and happiness.

Notes on pronunciation:

- *k* is soft, as in "king"
- *kh* is like the end of "kick," almost catching in the throat

Tones for the Mantra

HIGH							*Bha van*	
BASE		*kah*		*ta*		*no*		*tu*
LOW	*Lo*		*Sa mas*		*Sukhi*			

A VEDIC MANTRA TO COLLECT "SOUL POWER"

Taken from the *Eesha Upanishad,* this powerful mantra draws into the present moment all that our soul has strived for in its movement toward love, light, and truth. I use it often. I recommend using it whenever you feel disempowered or sucked into actions that you know will not lead to good results.

Kra-to Sma-ra Kru-tam Sma-ra

Translation: Oh my soul, remember past strivings, remember past strivings toward goodness and love.

Tones for the Mantra

This mantra can be sung in a hypnotic, cyclic arrangement of four variations using the three tones.

HIGH							
BASE	*Kra*	*to*	*Sma ra*	*Kru*	*tam*	*Sma*	*ra*
LOW							

HIGH		*to*					
BASE			*Sma ra*	*Kru*	*tam*	*Sma*	*ra*
LOW	*Kra*						

HIGH		*to*	*Sma ra*	*Kru*	*tam*	*Sma*	*ra*
BASE							
LOW	*Kra*						

HIGH							
BASE		*to*	*Sma*	*ra*	*Kru*	*tam*	*Sma*	*ra*
LOW	K*ra*							

VEDIC MANTRAS TO ACCOMPANY THE SUN SALUTATION (SURYA NAMASKAR)

THE FOLLOWING is a series of twelve Vedic mantras that are used in conjunction with the sun salutation, a flowing sequence of twelve connected yoga poses that is very popular in Hatha Yoga practice:

Om Mit-raa-ya Na-ma-ha
(We pay homage to the One who is the friend of all)

Om Ra-va-ye Na-ma-ha
(We pay homage to the Divine radiance)

Om Suur-yaa-ya Na-ma-ha
(We pay homage to the One who disperses darkness)

Om Bhaa-na-ve Namaha
(We pay homage to the One who diffuses light)

Om Kha-gaa-ya Na-ma-ha
(We pay homage to the One who travels in the sky)

Om Puush-Ne Na-ma-ha
(We pay homage to the One who nourishes all)

Om Hi-rań-ya-gar-bhaya Na-ma-ha
(We pay homage to that golden being who heals all things)

Om Ma-rii-cha-ye Na-ma-ha
(We pay homage to the Lord of the dawn)

Om Aa-dit-yaa-ya Na-ma-ha
(We pay homage to the One who is the child of the sky goddess)

Om Sa-vit-re Na-ma-ha
(We pay homage to the source of light and life)

Om Ar-kaa-ya Na-ma-ha
(We pay homage to the One who removes all distress)

Om Bhaas-ka-raa-ya Na-ma-ha
(We pay homage to the One whose brilliance leads to enlightenment)

Tone Pattern for All
of the Sun Salutation Mantras

HIGH				*ma*	
BASE	*Om Mit-raa*		*Na*		*ha*
LOW		*ya (go low for the syllable before Namaha)*			

VYAAHRITI MANTRAS

Vyaahriti means "utterance" or "declaration." The following Vedic mantras represent the seven planes of existence, associated with the seven chakras. The sounds of these mantras are a good contrast to the more feminine Tantric bijas detailed in appendix two. The mantras are written exactly the way they should be pronounced as individual utterances.

Om Bhu-hu
Om Bhu-va-ha
Om Su-va-ha
Om Ma-ha-ha
Om Ja-na-ha
Om Ta-pa-ha
Om Sat-yam

These seven mantras awaken the earth plane *(Bhur),* the heavenly plane *(Bhuvas),* that which is between earth and heaven *(Svaha),* the great plane of the Gods *(Mahat),** the many worlds beyond that *(Janah),* the realm of heat and spiritual fire at the heart of all existence *(Tapah),* and truth *(Satyam)* — the highest of all planes.

Notice that the first three mantras are the same as the first line of the sacred *Gayatri.* In the long form of the *Gayatri,* the entire sequence above is recited aloud, then a breath is inhaled through the left nostril. While the breath is held inside, the actual *Gayatri* is recited mentally. The *Gayatri* itself (without the vyaahritis) is a specific Vedic poetic meter, with three lines of eight syllables each:

* The Mahat is sometimes referred to as the mind of the universe.

Tat Sa-vi-tur Va-reh́-yam
Bhar-go De-vas-ya Dhi-ma-hi
Dhi-yo-yo-nah Pra-cho-da-ya-at

After recitation of the above three-line mantra, the breath is slowly released through the right nostril. This is a traditional practice of orthodox Hindus, performed as part of their Sandhya Upaasana and Sandhya Vandhana — morning and evening religious observances.

SANDHYA UPAASANA AND SANDHYA VANDHANA

THE FOLLOWING VEDIC mantras are Sandhya Vandhana (praise at the juncture hours of dawn and dusk), chanted as part of an elaborate sacred ritual Sandhya Upaasana (obligatory religious rite) that purifies the body and makes it a fitting temple for the indwelling spirit. Have some water available in a small cream pitcher or in a yogi's *lota* (*neti* pot), a water-holding device. For the first three mantras, pour some water into the palm of your right hand and sip it, as I will describe. For touching the body parts, use only your right hand. Note that there are other versions of this Sandhya Vandhana that make use of a slightly different set of mantras and gestures.

Om Ke-sha-vaa-ya Svaa-ha:
Sip water once after reciting the mantra

Om Maa-da-vaa-ya Svaa-ha:
Sip water once

Om Naa-raa-ya-naa-ya Svaa-ha:
Sip water once

Om Go-vin-daa-ya Na-ma-ha:
Wash both hands while reciting

Om Vish-ńa-ve Na-ma-ha:
Touch both nostrils, first right, then left, with index finger while reciting

Om Ma-du-suu-dha-naa-ya Na-ma-ha:
Touch both eyelids with ring finger (same as above)

Om Tri-vik-ra-maa-ya Na-ma-ha:
Touch both ears with little finger, as above

Om Vaa-ma-naa-ya Na-ma-ha:
Place center of palm on navel

Om Shree-dha-raa-ya Na-ma-ha:
Place center of palm on solar plexus

Om Hri-shi-kay-shaa-ya Na-ma-ha:
Place center of palm on crown of head

Om Pad-ma-naa-bhaa-ya Na-ma-ha:
Touch right shoulder with middle finger

Om Daa-mo-da-raa-ya Na-ma-ha:
Touch left shoulder with middle finger

TONE PATTERN FOR THE FIRST THREE MANTRAS

HIGH				
BASE	*Om-Ke-sha-vaa*	*ya*		*ha*
LOW			*Svaa*	

Tone Pattern for the Remaining Nine Mantras

HIGH				*ma*	
BASE	*Om Go-vin-daa*		*Na*		*ha*
LOW		*ya (or the syllable before Namaha)*			

The significance of each finger is explained in appendix two, under "Mudras of the Hands." All the above twelve mantras are associated with Vishnu, preserver of the universe. They are translated as follows:[1]

Keshava means "radiant one" or "long-haired one." Hair is associated with soul substance, which is why orthodox Hindus retain a long tuft from the crown of the head.

Maadhava: *Ma* is "learning." *Ma* is also Lakshmi, the goddess of wealth. This mantra honors Vishnu as the beloved of Lakshmi.

Naaraayana: *Naraah* means "derived from primeval waters," the source of all life; *ayana* is the abode of the creator who moves upon the waters and periodically renews the universe. (*Naraayana* is also translated as "the perfect one.")

Govinda: *Go* is cow; *Govinda* is Lord of the cows. Symbolically, Vishnu is being honored here as the provider of all nourishment.

Vishńave: Salutations to Vishnu, one who pervades and preserves the universe.

Madusoodhanaaya: Literally, "slayer of the demon Madhu." In Hindu mythology, Madhu is a demon born of the ear wax of Vishnu. Madhu also means "honey" and is associated with healing. It is interesting that the eyes, and not the ears, are touched for this mantra. Perhaps the mystical interpretation of the mantra's function in this ritual is that improper hearing can cloud our spiritual vision.

Trivikramaaya: One who encompasses the whole universe in three strides.

Vaamana: One of the incarnations of Vishnu as a dwarf who explodes into an immense being who crosses the world in three strides *(trivikrama).*

Shridaraaya: One who holds *Shri* in his or her heart. *Shri* is another name for Lakshmi, the goddess of wealth and prosperity.

Hrishikesha: The word *Hrishi* refers to the rays of light from the sun and the moon. This mantra honors Vishnu as lord of the senses, who brings us pleasure and happiness in life.

Padmanaabha: *Padma* is "lotus," *naabhi* is "navel." Brahma, the creator of the universe, is said to have sprung from Vishnu's navel. This mantra recognizes the purity of the abdomen and honors the belly as a source of creative energy.

Daamodhara: The rope-like power of the Divine, which binds us to itself like an umbilical cord binds a child to its mother.

APPENDIX 2

SHAKTI YOGA: TANTRIC MANTRAS

ASHWINI MUDRA: MUSCULAR CONTRACTION

The word "mudra" means "seal." Mudras, which are usually sacred gestures of the hands (see the end of this appendix for descriptions), are a way of configuring the body's energy circuitry. They are sometimes performed by muscle contractions, as in this case, which employs the two anal sphincter muscles located in the rectum.

The Ashwins are twin male gods of the morning — eternally young, handsome, and athletic, all qualities sought by yogis. In Hindu mythology, the Ashwins are physicians to the gods as well as horsemen known for their goodwill toward humans. The Sanskrit word for horse, *ashwa,* is a double entendre on the name of the mudra because yogis noticed that horses, greatly appreciated for their strength, have tremendous control over their anal muscles. In Kundalini or Shakti Yoga, the anal sphincters govern the root chakra, helping release primal energy into this first vortex. Perform this mudra before you begin chanting the chakra bijas.

The Method

Sit comfortably in your meditation posture (see chapter twelve for suggestions). Gently contract the anal sphincters. Hold for a count of three, sealing off the anal opening, then release gradually. Be present to the experience, and you will perceive an unfolding of energy like the opening of a flower each time you release the held contraction of the mudra.

BIJA MANTRAS OF THE SEVEN CHAKRAS

Use each of the following mantras, either seven or twenty-one times in rapid succession, employing a quick intake of breath after each utterance. These mantras are best recited internally. They may also be spoken aloud, but not sung. Concentrate on each chakra while you sound the mantra in the appropriate region or center of reference. When you complete the cycle, sit still and maintain an alert awareness of your body's energy field, taking in all the vibratory sensations that manifest inside your body, in your skin, and in the charged atmosphere immediately outside your body's physical form.

The mantras all sound like the drink "rum": *Rum* as in "rummy," *Yum* as in "yummy," *Hum* as in "humming." Do not pronounce *lam* as in "lamb" or "alarm." It should be pronounced like the "lum" in "alumni." *Vam* rhymes with the others ("vum").

Lam: I am (or have become) the earth. This bija is associated with the root chakra. Place your tongue on your upper palate to pronounce the mantra. Concentrate on the anal opening.

Vam: I am the cosmic waters. This bija is associated with the sexual chakra. Place your upper teeth inside your lower lip to pronounce the sound with a buzzing. Concentrate slightly above the genitals.

Ram: I am fire. This bija is associated with the power chakra in the abdomen. Roll the tip of your tongue on your upper palate to pronounce the mantra. Concentrate on your navel.

Yam: I am air. This bija is associated with the solar plexus. Separate your upper and lower teeth slightly, push the tip of your tongue toward your teeth, and pronounce the mantra.

Ham: I am space. This bija is associated with the throat chakra. Open your jaws wide to pronounce it.

Om: I am all that is. This bija is associated with the third eye, located in the space between the eyebrows in the center of the forehead. Whisper this mantra softly.

Silence: I am all that is and all that is not. The absence of produced sound is associated with the crown center.

KECHARI MUDRA: MUDRA OF THE TONGUE

THIS IS AN EXCELLENT YOGA mudra to use after the sequence of chakra bijas just described. *Kechari Mudra* is sometimes referred to as the "king of yoga mudras." It is performed by curling the tongue upward and backward, moving it up to the roof of the mouth and pushing it back as far as comfortable. Care must be taken not to injure the tendon that attaches your tongue to the bottom of your mouth.

Kriya yogis, the lineage of Paramahamsa Yogananda, state that the force that is rising upward in the body flows off the end of the tongue, like flames. Here a final connection is made. This mudra causes the pineal gland to vibrate by exciting the pituitary; the energy from these two forces, naturally drawn to each other, unites in the region between the eyebrows, awakening the third eye of unitive vision.[1]

BIJA MANTRAS TO EMPOWER THE SOUL

THE FOLLOWING BIJAS may be used in their pure form — *hoom, aim, gam,* and so on — for maximum potency. Sit in your favorite meditation position (see chapter twelve) and place your hands in a reverential gesture to chant these mantras. Move between making an external sound (vacaka), a whisper (upaamsu), and a sounding in the heart (maanasa). Inhale deeply after each utterance. Sit quietly when you are finished.

If uttered, say these mantras clearly and in articulate continuity, without rushing them or slurring the syllables into one another. They have been hyphenated in order to help you visually break down the syllables with ease. Remember to apply all the rules of pronunciation presented in appendix one to all the mantras in these subsequent appendixes.

To use these bija mantras devotionally, and to soften their effect, use *Om* before the mantra and *Namaha* after it. As explained in chapter eight, this adds a "time-release" or "buffered" effect to the power to the mantra.

Another variation combines the bija of a particular deity with the name of the deity. This is a powerful form, which can also be sung. The tones are easy, as indicated by the grids that follow. This third variation, which includes the name of the deity, may also be written in a dedicated mantra notebook, a practice known as *likhita japa,* or "writing mantras." Set an objective of writing 108 or 1,008 mantras; recite them clearly in your mind, or whisper them, as you write. You don't have to complete writing them all in a single sitting.

On special days of retreat, you may use a single mantra for a whole day, reciting it aloud, whispering it, writing it, or saying it in your mind. Otherwise, set a time period, say seven or twenty-one minutes, and write or recite for that amount of time. You may also recite these mantras using maala beads.

Hoom: Varma bija; embodys the energy of Shiva. Use it when tired or eager to infuse strength and stability into your soul.

The pure sound: *Hoom*

Devotional variation: *Om Hoom Na-ma-ha*

Sung variation: *Om Hoom Shi-vaa-ya Na-ma-ha*

The following tonal structure can be applied to all these mantras:

HIGH							*ma*	
BASE	*Om*	*Hoom*	*Shi*	*vaa*		*Na*		*ha*
LOW					*ya (go low for the syllable before Namaha)*			

Aim: Bija of Saraswati, the goddess of wisdom and learning. Use this mantra to remove mental blocks and to awaken creativity.

The pure sound: *Aim*

Devotional variation: *Om Aim Na-ma-ha*

Sung variation: *Om Aim Sa-ras-wa-ta- ye Na-ma-ha*

Gam: Bija of Ganesh. (Sounds like chewing gum.) Use it to remove obstacles in life and at the beginning of new undertakings.
The pure sound: *Gam*
Devotional variation: *Om Gam Na-ma-ha*
Sung variation: *Om Gam Ga-na-pa-ta-ye Na-ma-ha*

Kshroum: Bija of *Narashima,* the combined energy of the human and animal realms. Use it to remove fear.
The pure sound: *Kshroum*
Devotional variation: *Om Kshroum Na-ma-ha*
Sung variation: *Om Kshroum Na-ra-shim-haa-ya Na-ma-ha*

Kleem: Bija of *Kaamadeva.* Use it when lethargic or disinterested in life to awaken passion and bring satisfaction into your life.
The pure sound: *Kleem*
Devotional variation: *Om Kleem Na-ma-ha*
Sung variation: *Om Kleem Kaa-ma-de-vaa-ya Na-ma-ha*

Dum: Bija of Durga. Use it when situations are clouded over or darkened. This mantra dispels ignorance and channels a powerful light into those situations.
The pure sound: *Dum* (Sounds like "whom," but without prolonging the vowel; *avoid* saying it like "doom" as in "doomsday." Follow the pronunciation guide, placing the tip of your tongue between your teeth.)
Devotional variation: *Om Dum Na-ma-ha*
Sung variation: *Om Dum Dur-gaa-ya Na-ma-ha*

Shring: Bija of Lakshmi, the goddess of wealth. Use this mantra to generate abundance and to attract prosperity into your life.
The pure sound: *Shring*
Devotional variation: *Om Shring Na-ma-ha*
Sung variation: *Om Shring Ma-haa-laksh-mi-ye Na-ma-ha*

Kreem: Bija of Kali. Use it to dispel sorrow, to destroy negative thoughts and images, and to rid yourself of illness.

The pure sound: *Kreem*
Devotional Variation: *Om Kreem Na-ma-ha*
Sung Variation: *Om Kreem Ma-haa Kaa-li-ye Na-ma-ha*

Hreem: Bija of *Bhuvaneshwari,* mother of the universe. Use it for any purpose.
The pure sound: *Hreem*
Devotional Variation: *Om Hreem Na-ma-ha*
Sung Variation: *Om Hreem Bhu-va-nesh-wa-ri-ye Na-ma-ha*

SOME POPULAR TANTRIC MANTRAS

THE FOLLOWING TANTRIC mantras have a devotional quality, so they are often sung. The first mantra is popular in yoga studios across America; the third is a special variation of the same. The other mantras are not common to most Western yoga practitioners, but they are well-known among Tantric initiates and Shakti worshippers in India.

Om Na-mah Shi-vaa-ya

Translation: We worship the dance of energy that is creation.

Direction: Use *Om Na-mah Shi-vaa-ya* to deal with strong changes in your life, or simply to celebrate life in all its fullness. It is also a wonderful mantra for developing detachment from worldly concerns, infusing the yogi with inspiration toward spiritual pursuits.

Om Aa-di Pa-raa Shak-ti-ye Na-ma-ha

Translation: We offer praise to the primal, feminine energy that is the matrix of the universe.

Direction: Use *Om Aa-di Pa-raa Shak-ti-ye Na-ma-ha* to create a powerful force-field around you, especially in times of danger. You may also use it to protect your loved ones, visualizing their physical form as you chant the mantra.

Om Na-mah Shi-vaa-ya, Shi-vaa-ya Na-mah Om

Translation: We worship the dance of creation; may it dance itself through us.

Direction: Use this mantra palindrome to churn psychic toxicity out of your body, your place of work, your home, or a relationship. This particular variation will get the energy in your chakras to swirl around, so be prepared for strong sensations to arise in your awareness.

Om Hreem Shreem Kreem Pa-ra-maesh-wa-ri-ye Svaa-ha

Translation: The first three bijas belong to three powerful forms of Shakti: the Earth mother Bhuvaneshwari, the goddess Lakshmi, and Kali. Para, as you know, means "great"; *Ishwari* is the feminine form of addressing the goddess as ruler of the cosmos. This very sacred mantra summons the immensity of all the feminine energy that is available in the universe.

Direction: This is the root mantra of Devi, the supreme goddess. It is good to use this mantra in a ritualistic manner by offering leaves, flower petals, milk, or turmeric to a form of the goddess that you are most in tune with. Use this mantra conscientiously: its power is greatly venerated among Tantrics and believed capable of obtaining any type of result.

Om Shak-ti, Om Shak-ti, Om Shak-ti Om
Aa-dhi Shak-ti, Ma-haa Shak-ti, Pa-raa Shak-ti, Om

Translation: We praise Divine energy in all its forms; she is primal, great, and supreme.

Direction: Use this mantra in a standing position with your hands joined all the way above your head in the namaste gesture, arms straight up. This mudra is reserved for use when we want to bring ourselves into conscious awareness of the most high and to raise our energy all the way to the top of our head. Use this mantra to revive energy in your body, your mind, or in any situation or relationship that is losing energy. Stomp your feet while chanting the mantra, visualizing any negativity draining out through your feet and into the earth.

Kaa-li, Kaa-li, Ma-haa Maa-ya, Na-mo Kaa-li-ke Na-mo Na-ma-ha

Translation: We honor Kali for her ability to create the illusion of this world of forms. By her grace this veil will be removed, and we will directly behold the glorious vision of Divine presence.

Direction: Use this mantra when you are confused about what to do in a relationship or professional situation. Sit in your meditation posture (see chapter twelve), raise your palms above your head, interlace all fingers except the forefingers, which are stretched upward together to create a steeple-like effect. This mudra functions like a magic wand, dispelling any static that is interfering with your deepest perception.

MUDRAS OF THE HANDS, TO BE USED WITH MANTRA PRACTICE

MANY SPIRITUAL TRADITIONS around the world claim that there is a tremendous flow of energy in our hands. In yoga, each finger represents one of the five elements:

Elements Associated with the Fingers

thumb	*agni* (fire)
forefinger	*vaayu* (air)
middle finger	*akasha* (ether)
ring finger	*prithvi* (earth)
little finger	*jala* (water)

The fingers are also associated with the planets:

Planets Associated with the Fingers

index finger	Jupiter
middle finger	Saturn
ring finger	Uranus and the sun
little finger	Mercury
thumb	your personal energy field that makes contact with the energy of the planets through the mudra configurations

The fingers are also associated with the gunas, or aspects of nature:

Gunas Associated with the Fingers

thumb	*Paramaatma,* the Divine or cosmic soul
index finger	*jiva,* the individual soul
middle finger	*sattva* (purity)

ring finger	*rajas* (activity)
little finger	*tamas* (inertia)

Yoga mudras make use of special gestures involving the fingers to create specific circuits of energy in our spiritual and physical bodies, connecting us with the energy of the universe.

Four Mudras of the Hands

The following four mudras are powerful gestures that can accompany your mantra recitations, especially in Shakti Yoga:

Giṇana mudra: *Gnana* means "wisdom." (This ṇ is pronounced like the "n" in "singe" or "ginger.") For this mudra, touch the tip of the index finger to the tip (or middle) of the thumb to stimulate sacred knowledge and spiritual understanding.

Shani mudra: *Shani* is the name for the planet Saturn. In this mudra, connect the tip of the middle finger with the tip of the thumb to confer patience and facilitate purity of intention.

Soorya mudra: *Soorya* is the sun. For this mudra, connect the tip of the ring finger with the tip of the thumb to increase health and vitality.

Buddhi mudra: *Buddhi* is the intellect. For this mudra, touch the tip of the little finger to the tip of the thumb to enhance clarity. This is a great gesture for improving communication.

APPENDIX 3

BHAVA YOGA: BHAKTI MANTRAS

I recommend that you sing the following Sanskrit devotional phrases for your Bhava Yoga ritual, or simply as a devotional meditation. Each of these twenty-one mantras represents a quality of the Divine that we seek in our own soul. They can be recited one after the other, as in a litany, or you may take a single mantra and chant it twenty-one times, 108 times, or for a duration of twenty-one minutes. Chanting them all together in a sequence is extremely powerful.

Choose at least two tones: one high and the other low. Using three tones is ideal. I have provided a couple of traditional variations for your reference. Notice the emotional difference between saying these mantras and singing them. If you have any initial resistance, you can get past it by telling yourself that you will be singing for God. A whole world of spiritual emotion will open up for you.

DEVOTIONAL MANTRA LITANY

PRONUNCIATION REVIEW:

- Follow all the rules mentioned in previous appendixes, particularly remembering to place the tip of your tongue between your teeth to pronounce the underlined letters *t̲, d̲,* and *n̲*.
- Remember, ņ is to be pronounced like the "n" in "singe" or "ginger."
- ń is pronounced by curling the tongue upward, into the middle of the upper palate, as in the word *earn*.
- n̲ is to be pronounced with tip of tongue lightly against tip of teeth.
- ṇ is to be pronounced like the "n" in "king" or "lung" — in the back of the throat. (This will be introduced soon.)
- *n* is a normal English "n."
- Unless the vowel is doubled, such as "aa," don't prolong its sound; when doubled, don't extend it for too long — just twice the normal time.
- Finally, emphasize and aspirate all consonants followed by an *h*.

Use the tones as follows:

HIGH		*–tre (the last syllable of the main mantra before N̲amaha)*			
BASE	*Om Shri Maa*				*ha*
LOW			*N̲a*	*ma*	

Or, as a variation:

HIGH				*ma*	
BASE	*Om Shri Ma-haa-raaj ņi*		*N̲a*		*ha*
LOW		*–ye (syllable before N̲amaha)*			

1. *Om Shri Maa-t̲re N̲a-ma-ha* (Holy Mother, we adore you)
2. *Om Shri Ma-haa-raaj- ņi-ye N̲a-ma-ha* (Holy Queen, we adore you)
3. *Om Bhad̲-ra-muur-t̲i-ye N̲a-ma-ha* (Lover of benevolence, we adore you)

4. *Om Bhak-ta-pri-yaaa-ye Na-ma-ha* (Lover of devotees, we adore you)
5. *Om Bhak-ti-gam-yaa-ye Na-ma-ha* (Won by devotion, we adore you)
6. *Om Bha-yaa-pa-haa-ye Na-ma-ha* (Dispeller of fear, we adore you)
7. *Om Shar-ma-daa-yin-ye Na-ma-ha* (Giver of happiness, we adore you)
8. *Om Saad-vi-ye Na-ma-ha* (Of unequalled virtue, we adore you)
9. *Om Ni-raṇ -ja-naa-ye Na-ma-ha* (Unstained, we adore you)
10. *Om Nir-le-paa-ye Na-ma-ha* (Free from impurity, we adore you)
11. *Om Nir-ma-laa-ye Na-ma-ha* (Free from blemish, we adore you)
12. *Om Nish-kaa-maa-ye Na-ma-ha* (Free from desire, we adore you)
13. *Om Nit-ya-shud-daa-ye Na-ma-ha* (Ever pure, we adore you)
14. *Om Nit-ya-bud-dhaa-ye Na-ma-ha* (Ever wakeful, we adore you)
15. *Om Nir-ma-daa-ye Na-ma-ha* (Free from pride, we adore you)
16. *Om Ma-da-naa-shin-ye Na-ma-ha* (Destroyer of pride, we adore you)
17. *Om Nir-ma-maa-ye Na-ma-ha* (Free from thought of self, we adore you)
18. *Om Paa-pa-naa-shin-ye Na-ma-ha* (Destroyer of sin, we adore you)
19. *Om Duk-kha-han-tri-ye Na-ma-ha* (Taking away sorrow, we adore you)
20. *Om Su-khap-pra-daa-ye Na-ma-ha* (Conferring happiness, we adore you)
21. *Om Sar-va-shak-ti-maa-ye Na-ma-ha* (All powerful, we adore you)

SIMPLE KIRTANS

KIRTANS ARE the call-and-response chants that make the musical experience of Bhava Yoga accessible to everyone. Through their simple, evocative melodies, these repetitive chants quickly open our heart and flood our nervous system with loving energy. Each line is sung once by the caller, and the group responds identically. The same line can also be sung in other musical variations, requiring the responding group to listen intently in order to replicate the musical sequence. This causes the mind to become still and free from discursive thinking; it is hard to think while you listen in view of repeating both words and tune, then sing from the memory of that absorption.

The next line is played with in the same way, then both lines are put together and sung in a single melodic sequence that is repeated by the group.

Na-mah Dur-gaa-ye, Shree Kaa-li Maa
Na-mah Dur-gaa-ye, Na-mah Dur-ga

Translation: We worship you, fierce and blinding light of the goddess Durga — you who are also Kali, the mother of all beings.

Shree Ma, Kaa-li Ma, Aa-di Maa, Paa-hi Ma

Translation: We honor you, Mother Kali; your power is primal and you are indeed holy.

Ha-ra Ha-ra Ma-haa De-va Sham-bo
Kaa-shi Vish-wa-naa-tha Gaṇg-gay

Translation: All praise to you, great Lord of the universe. You, who make your home in Kashi by the river Ganges, are the living source of our joy.
Note on pronunciation: The letter *ṇ* (in *Gaṇg-gay)* is to be pronounced like the "n" in "king" or "lung" — in the back of the throat.

Aru-naa-cha-la Shi-va, Aru-naa-cha-la Shi-va
Aru-naa-cha-la Shi-va, Aru-naa-cha-la

Translation: We praise you, Shiva — you who dwell in the holy mountain of Arunachala, which represents the incarnation of your formless essence upon this earth.

TRADITIONAL VAISHNAVA MANTRAS

Om Na-mo Bha-ga-va-te Vaa-su-de-vaa-ya

Translation: We worship you, beloved, as the one who is goodness personified in divinity.

Shree Krish- ńa Sha-ra-nam Ma-ma

Translation: My refuge is the Lord Krishna.

Ha-ri Om

Translation: We offer our praise to you, Lord Hari (Vishnu). (*Hari* represents the energy essence of Brahman.)

Kleem Krish- ńaa-ya Go-vin-daa-ya
Go-pi-ja-na Val-la-bhaa-ya Svaa-ha

Translation: *Gopala* is a name for Krishna as cowherd, *Go* meaning "cow." *Gopijana* refers to him as the beloved of the cowherd girls, known as *gopis.* Mystically, all human souls are gopis who are drawn to the Divine like moths to a flame. In this Divine love, we are consumed and transformed. Notice that *Kleem,* the Tantric bija associated with Kama the God of love and passion, is a sort of Hindu cupid and a form of Krishna, who is the ultimate lover. *Govinda* is the protector of cows; Vishnu is the protector and provider of all human subsistence, which includes food.

Om Shreem Hreem Kleem Shree Krish- ńaa-ya Shree Go-vin-daa-ya
Shree Go-pi-ja-na Val-la-bhaa-ya Shreem Shreem

Translation: The above is a variation on the previous eighteen-syllable mantra, and is known as the *Siddha Gopala* mantra. A *siddha* is a yogi with tantric powers. Obviously, the Tantric influence is even stronger here than in the previous variation, with the additions of *Shreem* — the bija of Lakshmi — and *Hreem,* to dispel illusion, together with honorific addresses to each mantra. *Shree* is a title of respect which means "Your Holiness."

Om Na-mo Naa-raa-ya-naa-ya

Translation: "Naaraayana" is a name for Vishnu. *Naara* represents the primeval waters of creation; *Ayana* means "resting place" or "support."

Vishnu is the preserver of the universe, and is thus known as Naaraayana, the resting place and support of all creation. There are two forms for using this mantra. The above eight-syllable *(astaakshari)* form, which includes the syllable *Om,* is necessary to obtain *moksha* (liberation). For material gain and worldly problems, the *Om* is omitted:

Na-mah Naa-raa-ya-naa-ya

APPENDIX 4

NADA YOGA: TONES, PRACTICES, AND MEDITATIONS

BRAHMARI MUDRA: THE BUZZING YOGI

The objective of this practice is to open to your inner ear and listen to the inner sounds of your body.

1. Sit comfortably in your meditation posture (several options are listed in chapter twelve) and gradually — as though in slow motion — bring your hands toward your face.
2. Use your thumbs to press the *tragus* (the pointed flap of cartilage that lies above the earlobe, partially covering the entrance to the ear passage) against your ear canal to prevent sound from entering your ears. Next, shut your eyelids and use your index and middle fingers to prevent light from entering your eyes. These aperture-closings are known as "locks." Position your ring fingers so that their tips are lightly touching each nostril; they are kept ready so that you can press them against your nostrils and prevent air from entering or leaving your lungs. You are now controlling six

openings: a pair each of eyes, ears, and nostrils. This is known as the "six-way seal."

3. Raise your elbows high so that your forearms are at shoulder height, with your armpits wide open. Take a few moments to adjust your overall body posture and hold it steady. It is normal to hear a lot of rustling in your ears, but this will lessen considerably as you learn to hold still. Ignore your thoughts and listen intently to your body.
4. Take slow deep breaths. On the exhalations, allow yourself to hum in a relaxed way. There is no need to make it sound beautiful; just modulate your breathing so that the sound, coupled with the breath, is smooth and effortless. The idea is to imitate the buzzing of a bee, which is what the word *brahmari* means.
5. Hum for seven to twelve breaths, then inhale deeply and hold the air inside by blocking off your nostrils. Try to keep your mind empty of thoughts and images while you listen intently to the silence inside your body. Don't excessively prolong the retention of your breath; you should be able to release your breath smoothly when you exhale. During exhalation, slowly remove your hands from the blocked apertures, bringing them to rest comfortably on your knees or thighs.

Immediately following the release of the mudra, you will experience a tremendous spaciousness and a corresponding silence. Attune yourself to this silence and spaciousness. To progress into deeper levels of silence, repeat the locks, the humming, and the breath retention.

NADI SODHANA: THE PURIFYING BREATH

Nadi Sodhana is an exercise used in Nada Yoga to purify the solar and lunar channels, ida and pingala, that conduct hot and cold energy on either side of the spinal cord. Following brahmari, the yogic buzzing, Nadi Sodhana cleanses the central susumna nadi and distributes and balances energy in the chakras, creating a condition of calm and poise. As you learned in chapter eight, "Shakti Yoga," the nadis are psychic meridians that distribute prana — vital energy and life force — throughout our spiritual nervous system. The susumna is the central meridian that runs alongside the spinal cord.

1. Sit in your meditation position. Place your left palm on your left knee and position the fingers of that hand in the gnana mudra: thumb touching index finger. A variation of gnana mudra that I suggest for this practice is performed by pressing the tip of the forefinger against the base of the thumb and relaxing the other fingers, which are pointing downward. For your right hand, the tips of the forefinger and middle finger rest gently against the palm; keep the ring and little fingers aligned with each other. Curve the thumb toward the ring and little fingers so that it looks like a sort of clip, or a pair of horns on a bull. Hold this hand up to your face, palm facing you, and position it immediately in front of your nostrils so that the thumb can control the right nostril and the ring finger can control the left.

2. Using your thumb, block off your right nostril and inhale slowly and deeply through the left. Send your breath into your abdomen first, then continue inhaling into the upper portions of your lungs. Remember to breathe audibly, a type of sonic breathing I described in chapter thirteen *(ujjai pranayama)* and also on the accompanying audio tracks. Block off both nostrils by pressing your ring finger against your left nostril. Hold the breath inside for a count of three.

3. Open your right nostril and exhale slowly through it, expelling air from the upper part of your lungs first. Later in the exhalation, gently contract your abdominal muscles to empty your lower lungs. Block both nostrils and hold the breath outside for a count of two.

4. Open your right nostril and inhale slowly, relaxing the abdominal contraction and breathing into your lower lungs first to expand your abdomen; continue breathing into your

upper lungs. Block off both nostrils and hold the breath in for a count of three.

5. Breathe out slowly through your left nostril, upper lungs first, abdomen last. This completes one cycle. To repeat contiguous cycles, hold the breath out for a count of two by blocking both nostrils, then repeat the process from step one. To bring closure to the process, inhale through both nostrils smoothly and bring your right hand down to your right knee, positioning the fingers in gnana mudra, the same way your left hand is positioned. Exhale through both nostrils and rest.

Meditative Awareness During Nadi Sodhana

While inhaling through your left nostril, move your awareness from your left buttock upward, toward the left hemisphere of your brain. As you hold your breath inside, move your awareness from the left to the right hemisphere. Next, follow your exhalation down the right side of your body toward your right buttock. When you hold your breath outside, hold your awareness at the base of your spine. Then follow the breath upward from the right buttock along the right side of your body toward the right hemisphere of your brain as you inhale. As you hold your breath inside, move your awareness from the right to the left hemisphere of your brain. Finally, as you exhale, follow the breath down the left side of your body toward your left buttock. This completes one cycle.

TIPS: Breathe slowly and audibly. Coordinate and apply the same muscular contractions you did for the great yogic breath described in chapter fourteen. Sit still and relaxed while you engage in the process. Internally sound the *Om* with your exhalations; inhale in silence.

ASCENDING AND DESCENDING THE CHAKRAS

In these exercises, you will use the mantric syllables SA, RI, GA, MA, PA, DA, NI, and SA to ascend and descend the spine, vibrating each chakra with its appropriate musical syllable.

Method 1: For Those Who Don't Recognize Musical Pitches

You may use this method to develop an intuitive approach to your chakra frequencies by employing tones without regard to tempered tuning. The most important rule is to keep the tone steady, without wavering in pitch once you've started the tone. Try to resolve each tone smoothly. The great yogic breath described in chapter fourteen is the ideal breath cycle for this Nada Yoga meditation.

Start with a deep, low tone and sing out the syllable SA while maintaining an awareness of your root chakra, allowing your hips and spinal base to relax while the tone vibrates in that area, disintegrating any blockages and facilitating energy flow.

Next, use the syllable RI and raise the tone just a notch higher. Feel the shift in energy cause by the raised tone, and move your awareness into the space immediately above your pelvic area, relaxing your genitals and vibrating the tone in the second chakra for as long as your breath lasts.

In this manner, keep moving your pitch for each syllable: GA to your navel, MA to your heart, PA to your throat, DA to the point between your eyebrows, and NI to the crown of your head.

Once you have arrived at the crown chakra, reverse the process, singing SA on the same pitch you ended up with (or as high as you can go) for the crown chakra, then drop your pitch slightly to tone NI between your eyebrows. Likewise, incrementally drop your pitch for DA at your throat, PA at your heart, MA at your belly, GA above your genitals, and RI in the rectum.

The key to this process is to start at a very low note — as low as you can manage — then sense the right pitch for the next chakra, always moving higher in pitch as you ascend the spine. If you raise your pitch too high too fast, you will arrive at the highest register of your vocal range before you have gone through all the chakras. If you are overly cautious and use very short spaces between your tones, you will cover all your chakras within a narrow tonal range. The vision for this exercise is to know that the spectrum of your chakra vibrations lies within your vocal range.

Method 2: For Those Who Recognize Musical Pitches

In the second method, the body's energies are actually tuned to specific frequencies chosen for the chakras. As mentioned toward the end of chapter ten, many factors must be taken into consideration to balance and harmonize an individual's chakras, including such things as body type, time of day, place, and time of year. The following sequences are ones I've used in my own practice for many years, and they work really well for me. I offer them to you as a guideline; you can try them as recommended, then configure your own sequences based on your needs. You may refer to the Chakra Interval Chart provided after the practice to see how the intervals are positioned.

Tuning the Chakras

In this method, the energy released by moving between two frequencies activates the chakra. SA and RI function as a pair that governs the abdomen; the interval between the two activates the chakra. Similarly, the distance between GA and MA is used to activate the heart chakra, PA and DA to activate the throat, and NI and sa (higher octave) to activate the command center between the eyebrows.

The syllables ri and ga activate the seventh chakra, the crown center; they are represented in small letters because these tones are above the higher octave. Similarly NI and DA activate the second chakra, the sex center; they are underlined because they occur in the octave lower than the fundamental SA. To reach down to the root chakra, the lower octave PA and MA are utilized. The whole process spans a range of one-and-a-half octaves. You should be able to do this once you find a comfortable key to work with; if you can't, then slowly stretch yourself over time. This is how vocal exercises also become spiritual exercises.

There are three sequences of intervals that I recommend you work with; each is suggested for a specific time of day.

Between 4:00 A.M. and 11:00 A.M.:
RI (min 2nd); GA (maj 3rd); MA (reg 4th); DA (min 6th); NI (maj 7th)

Between 11:00 A.M. and 6:00 P.M.:

RI (maj 2nd); GA (min 3rd); MA (reg 4th); DA (min 6th); NI (min 7th)

Between 6:00 P.M. and 1:00 A.M.:

RI (maj 2nd); GA (maj 3rd); MA (augmented 4th); DA (maj 6th); NI (maj 7th)

Make sure you get some sleep between 1:00 A.M. and 4:00 A.M.!

SA, PA, and the octave "sa" are not written in the above sequences because they naturally occur in all of them. The first sequence is the Ashkenazi mode, often recognized in Middle Eastern music; the second is the Natural Minor, common in rock and pop; the third is known as the Lydian or Lesbian mode, favored in Indian music. In the key of C, their notes would occur as follows:

Ashkenazi mode: C, D-flat, E, F, G, A-flat, B, C
Natural Minor: C, D, E-flat, F, G, A-flat, B-flat, C
Lydian: C, D, E, F-sharp, G, A, B, C

The chart on the next page shows you how these intervals are spaced and where they will occur in the body.

CHAKRA INTERVAL CHART

INTERVAL	4:00 A.M. – 11:00 A.M.		11:00 A.M. – 6:00 P.M.		6:00 P.M. – 1:00 A.M.		CHAKRA
Maj 3rd	ga	e			ga	e	
Min 3rd			ga	e-flat			CROWN
Maj 2nd			ri	d	ri	d	
Min 2nd	ri	d-flat					
Octave	sa	c	sa	c	sa	C	
Maj 7th	NI	B			NI	B	COMMAND
Min 7th			NI	B-flat			
Maj 6th					DA	A	
Min 6th	DA	A-flat	DA	A-flat			
5th	PA	G	PA	G	PA	G	THROAT
Aug 4th					MA	F-sharp	
4th	MA	F	MA	F			
Maj 3rd	GA	E			GA	E	HEART
Min 3rd			GA	E-flat			
Maj 2nd			RI	D	RI	D	
Min 2nd	RI	D-flat					
ROOT	SA	C	SA	C	SA	C	ABDOMEN
Maj 7th	NI	B			NI	B	
Min 7th			NI	B-flat			
Maj 6th					DA	A	SEX CHAKRA
Min 6th	DA	A-flat	DA	A-flat			
5th	PA	G	PA	G	PA	G	
Aug 4th					MA	F-sharp	ROOT
4th	MA	F	MA	F			

PROGRAMS AND RESOURCES

In order to expand your vocabulary of mantras in each of the streams of Sound Yoga, I would like to recommend my three-CD *Yoga of Sound* program, which contains the titles *Shabda Yoga, Shakti Yoga,* and *Bhava Yoga.* To experience meditations in Nada Yoga, I recommend my CD *Nada Yoga*. For additional devotional chants using specific morning and evening ragas, try my two-CD set, *A.M. and P.M. Yoga Chants.* These programs are available nationwide, or through my Website, www.russillpaul.com. My Website will also give you information on Yoga of Sound events and special resources, such as my home study program.

YOGA OF SOUND AUDIO PROGRAMS PUBLISHED BY THE RELAXATION COMPANY

THESE CDs, also available individually, are a marvelous listening experience, crafted with great care and precision. Using world-class musicians and nature sounds recorded in the wild, these projects capture the authenticity of the streams of Sound Yoga you have learned about in this book. You can work with them in the privacy of your home or yoga studio.

Shabda Yoga

This program features Vedic mantras, starting with the simple *Om*. Each mantra is repeated in a call-and-response fashion so that you can listen and then chant along with the CD. There is also a powerful meditation called the *Rudram* from the *Yajur Veda*, which opens the album.

Shakti Yoga

This program features Tantric mantras to stimulate your energy system. *Om Namah Shivaya* and *Om Shakti* are fifteen-minute meditations. Also included is a raga meditation to open the chakras with the swara syllables.

Bhava Yoga

This program features a number of Bhakti mantras and various devotional movements that you can use while you chant. Vaishna mantras and Tantric devotional mantras to Kali and Shiva are also included.

Nada Yoga

This program features three long meditations, about eighteen minutes each, for use between twilight and midnight. You will be able to experience the subtle currents of energy possible through various Nada Yoga meditations and breathing practices.

A.M. & P.M. Yoga Chants

This excellent double album introduces you to a wide variety of devotional mantras and ragas for your morning and evening yoga and chanting practice. They are both in the Bhava Yoga category.

Three Levels of Study Using My Audio Products

There are three levels for working with these audio companions. First, you can just listen to them. You may even do this while you drive, listening to Shabda Yoga mantras on your way to work, Shakti Yoga during your midday break, Bhava Yoga on the way home, and Nada Yoga before you sleep. You can also use them as a backdrop for your yoga or meditation practice.

Second, you can learn mantras from these albums the way they're traditionally recited, allowing yourself to assimilate the power of their vibrations through proper pronunciation and inflection. These CDs have been tastefully arranged with both ancient and contemporary musical accompaniment that allows the mantras to feel accessible for the Western seeker, while remaining authentic in their delivery.

The third level is independence. You should eventually be able to produce the same effects that you encountered with these CDs through proper breathing technique and correct inflection and tones for the mantras. To achieve this, an ongoing study through workshops, retreats, seminars, and private study is recommended.

WORKSHOPS, RETREATS, AND SEMINARS

Workshops, retreats, and seminars help deepen and personalize the experience for you. Through these events, the various streams of Sound Yoga come alive and enter your body, mind, and heart through the physical immediacy of chanting in the same space with me. You will also get to interact with a learning community, then take home valuable tips and methods to incorporate into your practice.

Private Sessions

An intimate form of learning, this process allows for the maximum amount of energy and skill to be passed from teacher to student, a method practiced for many thousands of years in India. I recommend that a student first become well acquainted with my work and take at least one or two workshops with me before scheduling private sessions.

Home-Study Program

Because of my rigorous schedule, I am creating a home-study program that enables students to be guided in the privacy of their homes. The program will cover musical aspects of the Yoga of Sound tradition, mantra, and spiritual practices such as breathing and meditation.

Study Groups

Form your own dedicated learning community of about ten to twelve students, and pursue your Yoga of Sound experience together using the resources outlined in this chapter. If my schedule allows, I will be glad to spend some time with your group once or twice a year.

Pilgrimage

While it is always possible to learn mantras and Yoga of Sound practices through various means and resources in the West, there is a power and depth to encountering the raw, unmediated grandeur of this tradition in its own cultural and religious setting. Each year, my wife and I travel with a small group of pilgrims to South India, experiencing the ritualized used of mantras in ancient temples and ashrams. Should you feel the call to join us, you will also have the opportunity to study and practice mantra recitation with me in India in an informal setting.

LITERATURE

The following are books that I recommend for an in-depth understanding of Sound Yoga:

SONIC THEOLOGY: HINDUISM AND SACRED SOUND
by Guy L. Beck (Columbia, SC: University of South Carolina Press, 1993).
This is an excellent resource for understanding the traditional terminology of Sound Yoga and its historical development within the Hindu tradition. Guy is a respected ethnomusicologist and a dedicated musician, devoted to North Indian classical music.

THE WORLD IS SOUND, NADA BRAHMA: MUSIC AND THE LANDSCAPE OF CONSCIOUSNESS
by Joachim-Ernst Berendt (Rochester, VT: Inner Traditions Intl. Ltd., 1988).
Berendt had a great impact on the world of sound and spirituality, bringing together his vast experience of music with current findings in numerous branches of study, including physics, astronomy, biology, architecture, and mathematics.

SOUNDING THE INNER LANDSCAPE: MUSIC AS MEDICINE
by Kay Gardner (Stonington, MN.: Caduceus Publications, 1990).
The late Kay Gardner was both a musician and a healer. It is wonderful to have a woman's perspective on the subject, and she did a great job of combining information with practical exercises.

THE MYSTIC VISION: DAILY ENCOUNTERS WITH THE DIVINE
by Andrew Harvey and Anne Baring (San Francisco: Harper San Francisco, 1995).
This is a wonderful collection of mystical poetry and extracts from sacred texts, compiled by one of the most passionate mystics of our times, Andrew Harvey.

MEDITATION AS MEDICINE: ACTIVATE THE POWER OF YOUR NATURAL HEALING FORCE
by Dharma Singh Khalsa, M.D. (New York: Fireside Books, 2002).
This unusual medical doctor is also a yogi with a deep understanding of sacred sound and its use in the cure of physical ailments.

TOOLS FOR TANTRA
by Harish Johari (Rochester, VT: Inner Traditions of India, 1996).
Read Johari to understand the visual dimension of mantra known as yantra, as well as for a traditional view of Tantric mantra.

UNDERSTANDING MANTRAS
edited by Harvey P. Alper (Albany, NY: State University of New York Press, 1989).
A brilliant collection of essays and articles written by prominent researchers on the subject of mantra, including Andrew Padoux, Fritz Staal, and Ellison Banks Findley.

MUSIC AND MIRACLES
compiled by Don Campbell (Wheaton, IL: Quest Books, 1992).
Another excellent collection of essays and interviews on the subject of music and healing, including such luminaries as Dr. Jean Houston and Dr. Larry Dossey.

THE UPANISADS
by Juan Mascaro (London: Penguin Classics, Viking Press, 1965).
One of the most readable versions of the great breakthrough from the many to the one. Mascaro captures the essence of the sublime teachings of the Vedas in his selection of key passages from the principal Upanishads.

THE BHAGAVAT GITA
by Juan Mascaro (London: Penguin Classics, Viking Press, 1962).
A must-have for every postmodern yogi. The entire *Bhagavad Gita* is translated here into an eloquent flow of prose that captures the heart.

ENDNOTES

INTRODUCTION

1 Larry Dossey, M.D., *Meaning and Medicine: Lessons from A Doctor's Tales of Breakthrough and Healing* (New York: Bantam, 1992).

2 B.M. Dossey, L. Keegan, C.E. Guzzetta, and L.G. Koklmeier, *Holistic Nursing: A Handbook for Practice* (Rockville, MD: Aspen Publishers, Inc., 1988), quoted in Larry Dossey, *Meaning and Medicine.*

CHAPTER 1

1 James Haughton Woods, *The Yoga-System of Patanjali* (Delhi: Motilal Barnasidas Publishers, 1998).

2 Eckhart Tolle, *The Power of Now* (Novato, CA: New World Library, 1999).

3 Don Campbell, *The Mozart Effect: Tapping the Power of Music to Heal the Body, Strengthen the Mind and Unlock the Creative Spirit* (New York: Avon Books, 1997), p. 32.

4 Joachim-Ernst Berendt, *Nada Brahma, The World Is Sound: Music and the Landscape of Consciousness* (London: East West Publications, 1988), p. 136.

5 Candace B. Pert, *Molecules of Emotion: The Science Behind Mind-Body Medicine* (New York: Simon & Schuster, 1999).

6 See Don Campbell, *Music and Miracles* (Wheaton, IL: Quest Books, 1992), for essays and articles.

7 Allan D. Pierce, *Acoustics: An Introduction to Its Physical Principles and Applications.* (Acoustical Society of America Publications, 1989).

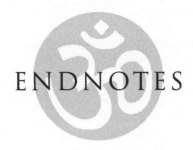

8 Hans Jenny, *Cymatics: A Study of Wave Phenomena and Vibration* (San Francisco: Macromedia Press, 2001).

9 Rupert Sheldrake, *A New Science of Life: The Hypothesis of Morphic Resonance* (Los Angeles: J.P. Tarcher, 1981).

10 Dharma Singh Khalsa, M.D., and Cameron Stauth, *Meditation as Medicine: Activate the Power of Your Natural Healing Force* (New York: Fireside Books, 2002).

11 Deepak Chopra, M.D., *Quantum Healing: Exploring the Frontiers of Mind-Body Medicine* (New York: Bantam, reprint edition, 1990).

12 Dorothy L. Retallack, *The Sound of Music and Plants* (Camarillo, CA.: DeVorss & Company, 1973).

13 *Deep in the Heart of the Tuva: Cowboy Music from the Wild East* (New York: Ellipses Arts, 1996). Book and CD.

14 Andrew Harvey and Ann Baring, *The Mystic Vision: Daily Encounters with the Divine* (San Francisco: Harper San Francisco, 1995).

CHAPTER 2

1 Andrew Harvey and Ann Baring, *The Mystic Vision: Daily Encounters with the Divine* (San Francisco: Harper San Francisco, 1995).

CHAPTER 3

1 George Ifrah, *The Universal History of Numbers: From Prehistory to the Invention of the Computer* (New York: John Wiley & Sons, Inc., 2000).

2 Joachim-Ernst Berendt, *Nada Brahma, The World is Sound: Music and the Landscape of Consciousness* (London and the Hague: East West Publications, 1988), p. 64.

3 Dharma Singh Khalsa, M.D., and Cameron Stauth, *Meditation as Medicine: Activate the Power of Your Natural Healing Force* (New York: Fireside Books, 2002).

CHAPTER 4

1 Eknath Easwaran, *Mantram Handbook* (India: Penguin Books, 1997).

2 Wayne Teasdale, *The Mystic Heart: Discovering a Universal Spirituality in the World's Religions* (Novato, CA.: New World Library, 2001).

CHAPTER 5

1 Kelley L. Ross, Ph.D., "Knowing Words in Indo-European Languages," copyright 2003, http://www.friesian.com/cognates.htm

2 Dr. K.L. Kamat, "Sir William Jones," December 12, 2003, http://www.kamat.com/kalranga/people/pioneers/w-jones.htm

3 Swami Rama, *Living with the Himalayan Masters: Spiritual Experiences of Swami Rama* (Honesdale, PA: Himalayan Institute Press, 1980).

4 Gary Zukav, *Seat of the Soul* (New York: Free Press, 1990 reprint edition).

5 Harvey P. Alper, *Understanding Mantras: SUNY Series in Religious Studies* (Albany, NY: State University of New York Press, 1989).

6 *Activate the Power of your Natural Healing Force* (New York: Fireside Books, 2002).

7 Alper, *Understanding Mantras.*

CHAPTER 6

1 Andrew Harvey and Ann Baring, *The Mystic Vision: Daily Encounters with the Divine* (San Francisco: Harper San Francisco, 1995).

2 Harvey P. Alper, *Understanding Mantras: SUNY Series in Religious Studies* (Albany, NY: State University of New York Press, 1989).

3 Juan Mascaro, *The Upanisads* (London: Penguin Books, 1965), p. 61.

CHAPTER 7

1 Hazrat Inayat Khan, *The Mysticism of Sound and Music* (Boston: Shambhala, 1996).

2 Wei Lian, "The Scientific Experiments on Water Crystals vs. the Origin and Elimination of Sickness," *Pure Insight*, June 2, 2003, http://www.pureinsight.org/pi/articles/2003/6/2/1626.htm

3 Santhigiri Ashram's Website, http://www.prodigyweb.net.mx/santhigi/guru/meaning.htm

4 Rama Prasada, translator, in Guy L. Beck, *Sonic Theology: Hinduism and Sacred Sound* (Columbia, SC: University of South Carolina Press, 1993).

5 William A. Graham, "Beyond the Written Word: Oral Aspects of Scripture in the History of Religion" in Beck, *Sonic Theology*, p. 65.

6 W. Norman Brown, "The Creative Role of the Goddess Vac in the *Rig Veda*" in Guy L. Beck, *Sonic Theology: Hinduism and Sacred Sound* (Columbia, SC: University of South Carolina Press, 1993), p. 394.

7 G.K. Bhat, "Vak in Satapatha Brahmana," in Beck, *Sonic Theology*.

8 John G. Cramer, "Sound of the Big Bang," November 10, 2003, http://faculty.washington.edu/jcramer/BBSound.html

9 Fritjof Capra, *The Tao of Physics* (Boston: Shambhala, 2000).

10 Robert Roy Britt, "The Music of Black Holes," April 9, 2002, Space.com, http://www.space.com/scienceastronomy/astronomy/blackhole_music_020409-1.html

11 Britt, "The Music of Black Holes."

12 Joachim-Ernst Berendt, *Nada Brahma, The World is Sound: Music and the Landscape of Consciousness* (London and the Hague: East West Publications, 1988), p. 66.

13 Don Campbell, *The Mozart Effect: Tapping the Power of Music to Heal the Body, Strengthen the Mind, and Unlock the Creative Spirit* (New York: Avon Books, 1997).

CHAPTER 8

1 Andrew Harvey and Ann Baring, *The Mystic Vision: Daily Encounters with the Divine* (San Francisco: Harper San Francisco, 1995), p. 111.

2 Hans Jenny, *Cymatics: A Study of Wave Phenomena and Vibration* (San Francisco: Macromedia Press, 2001).

3 Ashok Bedi, M.D., *Path to the Soul: The Union of Eastern and Western Wisdom to Heal Your Body, Mind, and Soul* (York Beach, MA: Samuel Weiser Inc., 2000).

4 Harish Johari, *Tools for Tantra* (Rochester, VT: Inner Traditions, 1986).

5 Wade T. Wheelock, "Mantra in Vedic and Tantric Ritual," in Harvey P. Alper, *Understanding Mantras* (Albany, NY: State University of New York Press, 1989), pp. 96-122.

CHAPTER 9

1 Guy L. Beck, *Sonic Theology: Hinduism and Sacred Sound* (Columbia, SC: University of South Carolina Press, 1993), p. 23.

2 "The Hare Krishna Mantra, 'There's Nothing Higher. . .': A 1982 Interview with George Harrison," copyright Bhaktivedanta Manor 2003, http://www.krishnatemple.com/manor/harrison

CHAPTER 10

1 George Leonard, *The Silent Pulse: A Search for the Perfect Rhythm That Exists in Each of Us* (New York: Bantam Books, 1981).

2 Robert Roy Britt, "The Music of Black Holes," Space.com, April 9, 2002, http://www.space.com/scienceastronomy/astronomy/blackhole_music_020409-1.html

3 Patanjali, *Yoga Sutras Part 1*: 27, 28.

4 Guy L. Beck, *Sonic Theology: Hinduism and Sacred Sound* (Columbia, SC: University of South Carolina Press, 1993).

5 Don Campbell, "Sound and the Miraculous: An Interview with Jean Houston," in Campbell, *Music and Miracles* (Wheaton, IL: Quest Books, 1992), pp. 9-17.

6 Pandit A. Mahadeva Sastri, "Yoga Upanisads," in Beck, *Sonic Theology,* p. 132.

7 T. R. Srinivasa Iyyengar, "The Yoga Upanisads" in Beck, *Sonic Theology,* p. 95.

8 Kahlil Gibran, *The Prophet* (New York: Alfred A. Knopf, 1923, 1966).

9 Rai Bahadur S. C. Vasu, "The Siva Samhita" in Beck, *Sonic Theology,* p. 103.

10 Pancham Sihn, "Hatha Yoga Pradipika" in Beck, *Sonic Theology,* p. 104.

11 Joachim-Ernst Berendt, *Nada Brahma, The World is Sound: Music and the Landscape of Consciousness* (London: East West Publications, 1988), p. 64.

12 Berendt, *Nada Brahma,* p. 61.

13 For an expanded understanding of vertical and horizontal music, see the author's article "In the Beginning Was Music" in Beatrice Bruteau, ed., *The Other Half of My Soul: Bede Griffiths and the Hindu-Christian Dialogue* (Wheaton, IL: Quest Books, 1996).

14 A.S. Panchapakesa Iyer, *Karnataka Sangeeta Sastra: Theory of Carnatic Music* (Madras, India: 1996).

15 Joachim-Ernst Berendt, *Nada Brahma,* p. 116.

16 Leonard, *The Silent Pulse.*

CHAPTER 11

1 Dharma Singh Khalsa, M.D., and Cameron Stauth, *Meditation as Medicine: Activate the Power of Your Natural Healing Force* (New York: Fireside Books, 2002), p. 4.

2 Juan Mascaro, *The Bhagavat Gita* (Great Britain: Penguin Books, 1962), p. 71.

3 Don Campbell, *The Mozart Effect: Tapping the Power of Music to Heal the Body, Strengthen the Mind, and Unlock the Creative Spirit* (New York: Avon Books, 1997), p. 39.

CHAPTER 12

1 Joachim-Ernst Berendt, *Nada Brahma, The World is Sound: Music and the Landscape of Consciousness* (London and the Hague: East West Publications, 1988), p. 81.

2 Matthew Fox, *Passion for Creation: The Earth-Honoring Spirituality of Meister Eckhart* (Rochester, VT: Inner Traditions International, 2000).

3 A.K. Ramanujan, *Speaking of Siva* (Great Britain: Penguin Books, 1973), p. 19.

4 Bede Griffiths, *Return to the Center* (Springfield, IL: Templegate Publishers, 1976).

5 Juan Mascaro, *The Upanisads* (Great Britain: Penguin Books, 1965), p. 61.

6 Psalm 24.

CHAPTER 13

1 Candace B. Pert, *Molecules of Emotion: The Science Behind Mind-Body Medicine* (New York: Simon & Schuster, 1999).

2 Soumy Ana, "Oxygen? What Do the Experts Say?" January 4, 2003, http://www.suite101.com/article.cfm/aerobics/96650

3 "Oxygen and Cancer," copyright 2004, http://www.alkalizeforhealth.net/oxygen.htm

4 Dr. Otto Warburg, "The Prime Cause and Prevention of Cancer," lecture delivered to Nobel Laureates on June 30, 1966, at Lindau, Lake Constance, Germany, http://www.alkalizeforhealth.net/Loxygen2.htm

5 "Nurse Bob's MICU/CCU Survival Guide," http://rnbob.tripod.com/

6 *Ibid.*

7 St. Benedict, "The Holy Rule of St. Benedict," 1949 Edition, translated by Rev. Boniface Verheyen, OSB of St. Benedict's Abbey, Atchison, Kansas, http://www.ccel.org/b/benedict/rule2/rule.html

8 Joachim-Ernst Berendt, *Nada Brahma, The World is Sound: Music and the Landscape of Consciousness* (London and the Hague: East West Publications, 1988), p. 35.

CHAPTER 14

1 Tools For Exploration, Inc., "The Healing Effect of Sound and Music," http://www.toolsforwellness.com/medhealing.html

2 John Cramer, "Sound of the Big Bang," audio file, http://www.npl.washington.edu/AV/BigBangSound_2.wav

3 John Cramer, "Sound of the Big Bang" article, November 10, 2003, http://faculty.washington.edu/jcramer/BBSound.html

4 Georg Feuerstein, "The Philosophy of Classical Yoga," in Guy L. Beck, *Sonic Theology: Hinduism and Sacred Sound* (Columbia, SC: University of South Carolina Press, 1993).

5 9 ways Mystery School of Shamanic Studies, "Hans Jenny," *Sacred Sound Tools,* copyright 2002, http://9waysmysteryschool.tripod.com/sacredsoundtools/id12.html

6 Kay Gardner, *Sounding the Inner Landscape: Music as Medicine* (Stonington, ME: Caduceus Publications, 1990), p. 120.

7 John Beaulieu, *Music and Sound in the Healing Arts* (Barrytown, NY: Station Hill Press, 1995).

8 Juan Mascaro, *The Upanisads* (Great Britain: Penguin Books, 1965), p. 102.

9 Georg Feuerstein, "Textbook of Yoga," in Beck, *Sonic Theology,* p. 26.

10 Nitin Kumar, "Om — An Inquiry into its Aesthetics, Mysticism, and Philosophy," Exotic India, December 2001, http://www.exoticindiaart.com/article/om

11 Mascaro, *The Upanishads,* p. 79.

CHAPTER 15

1 Annemarie Schimmel, *Mystical Dimensions of Islam* (Chapel Hill, NC: University of North Carolina Press, 1975).

2 Rosemary Cunningham, "Visiting a Sufi," *Spirituality & Health,* Fall 2001, http://www.spiritualityhealth.com/newsh/items/article/item_3617.html

3 The Canadian Society of Muslims, Toronto, http://muslim-canada.org/sufi/zikr5.htm

4 www.sacredcircles.com/THEDANCE/HTML/DANCEPAG/AAGLOSS/ZIKR.HTM

5 The Canadian Society of Muslims, Toronto, http://muslim-canada.org/sufi/zikr5.htm

6 Anonymous, *Meditations on the Tarot: A Journey into Christian Hermeticism,* translated by Robert Powell (Los Angeles: J. P. Tarcher, 2002).

CHAPTER 16

1 Joachim-Ernst Berendt, *Nada Brahma, The World is Sound: Music and the Landscape of Consciousness* (London: East West Publications, 1988), p. 5.

2 Pierre Sollier, "Biography [of Tomatis]," http://www.tomatis.com/English/Articles/Biography.html

3 To learn more about the Tomatis method, visit www.tomatis.com

4 Don Campbell, "Listening, The Ear, and Development: The Work of Dr. Alfred A. Tomatis," in *New Horizons for Learning,* http://www.newhorizons.org/spneeds/inclusion/information/campbell_d.htm

5 Campbell, "Listening, The Ear, and Development."

6 Emily Dickinson, *The Complete Poems of Emily Dickinson* (San Francisco: Back Bay Books, 1976).

7 Alfred A. Tomatis, *The Conscious Ear: My Life of Transformation Through Listening* (Barrytown, NY: Station Hill Press, 1992).

8 Peter Russell, *From Science to God: A Physicist's Journey into the Mystery of Consciousness* (Novato, CA: New World Library, 2003).

9 Russell, *From Science To God,* pp. 82-85.

10 Dr. James V. Hardt, "A Tale of Self-Discovery" in *Megabrain Reports,* May 1994, http://biocybernaut.com/publications/history.html

11 Rabindranath Tagore, *Songs of Kabir* (New York: Samuel Weiser, Inc., 1988).

CHAPTER 17

1 Juan Mascaro, *The Upanisads* (Great Britain: Penguin Books, 1965), p. 120.

EPILOGUE

1 Wayne Teasdale, *A Monk in the World: Cultivating a Spiritual Life* (Novato, CA: New World Library, 2002), p. 219.

2 Juan Mascaro, *The Upanisads* (Great Britain: Penguin Books, 1965), p. 61.

APPENDIX 1

1 Translations for these mantras were based on Margaret and James Stutley, *Harper's Dictionary of Hinduism* (San Francisco: Harper & Row, 1984) and V. Krishnamurthy, "Gems from the Ocean of Hindu through Vision and Practice," May 1, 1999, http://www.geocities.com/Athens/Rhodes/2952/gohitvip/1208page4.html

APPENDIX 2

1 The Arrya Mission, "Kechari Mudra," http://www.geocities.com/kriyadc/kechari.html

INDEX

Page numbers in boldface refer to mantras, exercises, and practices with specific instructions.

TRACK INFORMATION FOR YOGA OF SOUND AUDIO COMPANION

To download these MP3 audio tracks, visit www.russillpaul.com/download.html

I hope with these audio tracks to personally train you, and lead you to independence, in many basic practices and mantras of the Yoga of Sound. The program represents all the four major streams of Sound Yoga — Shabda Yoga, Shakti Yoga, Bhava Yoga, and Nada Yoga; the distinct types of mantras —Vedic, Tantric, and Devotional mantras; and the key elements of Sound Yoga — breath, movement, sound, posture, and consciousness.

For best results do not use headphones when working with these tracks as it will affect the accuracy of your pitch. Please read the section "Harmony and Attunement" on page 143 for more information about headphones and sound systems. Chapter 11, "Preparation and Mantra Shastra," provides valuable information that can be incorporated into your personal practice of Sound Yoga.

Each experiential track is preceded by a teaching track that verbally introduces you to the understanding, pronunciation, and practice of a particular exercise or mantra. The experiential tracks are all odd numbers, while the verbal, teaching tracks are even numbers. Focusing on the experiential tracks allows you to get deep into your practice without the explanations impinging on your experience. This separation, essentially between left and right brain learning, also allows you to program your MP3 player several different ways: 1) You can loop, or repeat, a particular practice or teaching so that you learn it deeply and thoroughly, 2) You can configure specific practices in sequences and combinations to suit your emphasis on a particular day or week, or 3) You can work with all the audio tracks, from start to finish, as a comprehensive workout in the Yoga of Sound.

For more extended chanting practice in mantras, I recommend my other audio programs with The Relaxation Company. See Programs and Resources on page 273.

1. Invocation to *Ganesh,* the remover of obstacles. A traditional Vedic mantra chanted in Vedic meter. Join palms at the heart and visualize all obstacles being removed from the flow of energy in your body. See page 78, "The Music of Shabda Yoga." (From The Yoga of Sound three-CD set, the Relaxation Company, © 2000. Used with permission.) (1:22)

2. Welcome and Introduction. (1:08)

3. *Om Namah Shivaaya* — exercise track — Here you will practice this Tantric, devotional mantra with music. See Appendix Two, page 254, for more explanation of the mantra. (2:27)

4. The vowel O — teaching track — Here I explain how to use this sound on the breath *(upamsu)* and how to incorporate movement into the sound. See page 192, "Circle of Power." (5:32)

5. Vowel O — exercise track — Learn to practice the sound with music. (3:32)

6. The universal mantra *Om* — teaching track — Explains how to pronounce the mantra externally. See Chapter 14, as well as "The Audible Breath" on page 166. (2:36)

7. The mantra *Om* — exercise track — Practice the mantra with music in the Tantric method. (2:36)

8. The Tantric bija *Hoom* — teaching track — Explains how this bija mantra associated with Shiva can be used with the *Shiva-Linga mudra* and breath work. See Appendix Two, pages 251 and 252. (1:35)

9. The mantra *Hoom* — exercise track — Practice the mantra with music. (0:59)

10. The Tantric bija *Aim* — teaching track — Explains how this Saraswati bija mantra can be used in combination with Anjali mudra and pranayama. See Appendix Two, page 251 and 252. (1:33)

11. The mantra *Aim* — exercise track — Practice the mantra *om aim namaha* with music. (1:45)

12. Vedic Mantra to Guide Us on the Path to Enlightenment — teaching track — Explains how to pronounce the sounds in this mantra sequence. See Appendix One, page 239 for words, pronunciation guidelines, and musical tones. (1:45)

13. Chanting *"Asato ma sadgamaya, tamaso ma jyotirgamaya, mrityorma amritamgamaya …"* with music. (1:28)

14. The Sacred *Gayatri* to Illuminate Our Meditations — teaching track — See Appendix One, page 241, for words, pronunciation guidelines, and musical tones. (1:36)

15. The *Gayatri* mantra — exercise track — Chant the sacred *Gayatri* with music: *Om bhur bhuvas svaha, tat savitur vareynam, bargo devasya dhimahi, dhyoyona prachodayaat.* (2:27)

16. A Vedic mantra to Heal Our Planet — teaching track — Explains how to pronounce the words in this pithy mantric prayer. (1:03)

17. Chanting *"Lokah samasta sukhino bhavanthu"* with music. (From The Yoga of Sound three-CD set, the Relaxation Company, © 2000. Used with permission.) (1:53)

18. Nada Yoga vocal technique — teaching track — Explains how musical tones can stimulate, balance, and heal the chakras. See Appendix Four, page 270, to understand this exercise. (3:10)

19. Nada Yoga practice — exercise track — Meditate on the tonal sequence and then sing along. See Chakra Interval Chart on page 272. (3:23)

20. Preparing to dance a mantra with Kali: *Shree Ma, Kali Ma, Aadhi Ma, Pahi Ma.* (2:49)

21. Dancing with the Dark Mother — A devotional kirtan to Kali, the matrix of creation and primal goddess. See "Simple Kirtans" in Appendix Three, page 262; also see "Blood of the Goddess" on page 82. (Music extracted from The Yoga of Sound three-CD set, the Relaxation Company, © 2000. Used with permission.) (3:00)

ABOUT THE AUTHOR

A native of Chennai (Madras City) in south India, Russill Paul took to playing stringed instruments at the early age of four and began playing professionally in his teens. In 1984, he underwent a powerful transition that motivated him to live as a monk under the late Dom Bede Griffiths, a pioneering Benedictine spiritual teacher and modern-day sage, who directed Shantivanam, a Hindu-Christian Ashram in south India. Here, Russill was able to bring together his ancestral Hindu heritage with his Christian upbringing.

During the five years he spent as a monk, Russill studied Sanskrit chanting and south Indian classical music, in addition to yoga, meditation, and philosophy. The most powerful component to his transformation was a series of profound spiritual experiences that affected his music and his education.

For almost twenty years, Russill has toured extensively in North America and internationally, presenting concerts, workshops, and seminars at conferences, spiritual centers, and retreat facilities. For more than fifteen years, he has taught in graduate (Masters in Liberal Arts) and postgraduate (Doctorate in Ministry) academic programs of Creation Spirituality nationwide. He began at the Institute in Culture and Creation Spirituality at Holy Names College in Oakland, California, and then proceeded to Naropa University Oakland and the University of Creation Spirituality in Oakland, and finally, Wisdom University of San Francisco, California.

Russill presently directs his students through his own spirituality-training program: a Yogic Mystery School that puts the power of technology to work to create the semblance of traditional training in the sacred knowledge of mantra, the spirituality of Indian music, and the power of yogic meditation. This is a distance-learning program that combines specialized resources with active student support through the internet, and this book is an invaluable resource to the training.

Russill has also been involved with the music industry for over two decades, recording professionally for movie soundtracks under well-known music directors in India and recording and producing a wide selection of his own world class, yoga-related recordings in the United States through The Relaxation Company, a leading publisher of healing music.

He lives with his wife in Austin, Texas. Together they conduct a special chanting pilgrimage and retreat in south India each year.

To learn more, contact Russill Paul through his website:
www.russillpaul.com

NEW WORLD LIBRARY is dedicated to publishing books and other media that inspire and challenge us to improve the quality of our lives and the world.

We are a socially and environmentally aware company, and we make every attempt to embody the ideals presented in our publications. We recognize that we have an ethical responsibility to our customers, our employees, and our planet.

We serve our customers by creating the finest publications possible on personal growth, creativity, spirituality, wellness, and other areas of emerging importance. We serve our employees with generous benefits, significant profit sharing, and constant encouragement to pursue our most expansive dreams. As members of the Green Press Initiative, we print an increasing number of books with soy-based ink on 100 percent postconsumer waste recycled paper. Also, we power our offices with solar energy and contribute to nonprofit organizations working to make the world a better place for us all.

Our products are available
in bookstores everywhere.
For our catalog, please contact:

New World Library
14 Pamaron Way
Novato, California 94949

Phone: 415-884-2100 or 800-972-6657
Catalog requests: Ext. 50
Orders: Ext. 52
Fax: 415-884-2199

Email: escort@newworldlibrary.com
Website: www.newworldlibrary.com